PRACTICING EXCELLENCE:
A PHYSICIAN'S MANUAL TO EXCEPTIONAL HEALTH CARE

"This is an excellent manual and should be required reading for all physicians, including medical students."
Floyd D. Loop, MD, Former CEO, Cleveland Clinic (1989-2004)
Studer Group Medical Advisor

"This is an amazing articulation of the secrets of the successful patient visit. Every provider, no matter how good, can benefit from Dr. Beeson's pearls."
David Spees, MD, Family Medicine Physician

"A very practical how-to guide. Addressed virtually all areas of push back!"
Steven Gabbe, MD, Dean, Vanderbilt University School of Medicine

*"Packed with valuable suggestions and tools that I can easily incorporate into my own practice as an individual physician.
I came away from this book inspired to be a leader..."*
Phil Yphantides, MD, Family Medicine Physician

"Extraordinary ideas."
Rick Gessner, Software Developer

D0179612

PRACTICING EXCELLENCE

A PHYSICIAN'S MANUAL TO EXCEPTIONAL HEALTH CARE

Stephen C. Beeson, MD

Medical care, workplace conditions,

clinical quality, service, and the culture of

a medical organization will ultimately

be determined by the conduct of its physicians.

TABLE OF CONTENTS

    The Physicians' Role
    Physician Change

    The Case for Service—Patient Compliance
    The Case for Service—Growth, Market Share, and Loyalty
    The Case for Service—Malpractice Risk
    The Case for Service—Physician Relationships to Staff
    The Case for Service—Physician Relationships to Colleagues

    The First Impression
    Exam Room Preparedness
    Techniques in History Taking
    The Physician Exam
    Providing Patient Information
    Patient/Physician Collaboration
    Patient Follow-up
    Effective Appointment Closure

FOREWORD

You are holding in your hands an important book, and one whose time has come.

When I wrote *Hardwiring Excellence: Purpose, Worthwhile Work, Making a Difference* back in 2003, my goal was to shine a light on what the nation's best hospitals are doing to create and sustain world-class organizations. My book offers a wealth of specific prescriptive tools and practices aimed at managers at all levels.

The book and its message were quite well received. It wasn't long before I started hearing comments like, "Quint, we love the way everyone, from our CEO to our nurses to our cafeteria workers, is changing the way they think about patient service. Now, what about our physicians? They're asking for a book, too!"

As it turned out, I didn't write that book. Dr. Beeson did! (And I believe that, as a physician, he is far more qualified to do the job.)

Practicing Excellence: A Physician's Manual to Exceptional Health Care is outstanding. It directly addresses the physician's role in living the principles that lead to organizational excellence. Written *by* a physician *for* physicians—and for all leaders who work *with* physicians—it is unlike any book I've seen in the marketplace.

I want to say up front that I have great admiration and respect for these men and women who move through the world healing patients and saving lives. And having spent years working with hospitals across America, I have met countless physicians. I know firsthand how central they are in the pursuit of outstanding health care.

When a hospital or medical group can get physicians to enthusiastically embrace an overarching, organization-wide mission to become a better place for employees to work, physicians to practice, and patients to receive care—well, that organization will be unstoppable in its pursuit of excellence.

That's what I believe Dr. Beeson's book can accomplish. When your organization uses it as a companion to *Hardwiring Excellence*, you will finally be able to get everyone "on the same page." Together, these two books are a powerful prescription for creating and sustaining world-class care.

As you'll see, *Practicing Excellence* provides the tools and practices physicians can use to decrease patient and family anxiety while increasing patient satisfaction and trust with their caregiver. It also addresses ways administrators can work with physicians to assure their full engagement and buy-in to the health care organization's mission.

Now, before you start reading, I would like to introduce and clarify a few of the concepts you will encounter in *Practicing Excellence*.

This is the Healthcare Flywheel℠. It shows how organizations can create momentum for change by engaging the passion of their employees to apply prescriptive actions guided by the Nine Principles® of Service and Operational Excellence to achieve bottom-line results. (Please note that you can read more about the Healthcare Flywheel in the excerpt from *Hardwiring Excellence* beginning on page 163 of this book.)

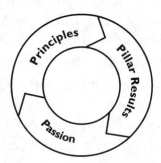

By continually reinforcing how daily choices and actions connect back to these core values at the hub of the Flywheel—purpose, worthwhile work, and making a difference—leaders will reinforce these behaviors and effect change more quickly.

The "Pillar Results" segment of the Flywheel refers to the Five Pillars that provide the foundation for setting organizational goals and direction for service and operational excellence. They are **People, Service, Quality, Finance,** and **Growth.**

The "Principles" segment refers to the Nine Principles of Service and Operational Excellence that provide a road map for achieving goals under the Five Pillars. The Nine Principles are:

1. Commit to Excellence

2. Measure the Important Things

3. Build a Culture around Service

4. Create and Develop Leaders

5. Focus on Employee Satisfaction

6. Build Individual Accountability

7. Align Behaviors with Goals and Values

8. Communicate at All Levels

9. Recognize and Reward Success

The "Passion" segment, of course, is self-explanatory. People in health care tend to be passionate and self-motivated by nature. But when a work culture is defined by too much emphasis on the negative, employees quickly become de-motivated.

In my work with hospitals, I teach leaders how to reignite that innate passion and get the Flywheel spinning in the right direction. (In some organizations, it's not just stalled; it's actually spinning backward!)

Once prescriptive to do's (which vary from organization to organization) are implemented, employees quickly see the results of their initial efforts: lower staff turnover, higher employee, physician, and patient satisfaction, improved service and quality, and a healthier bottom line. The Flywheel turns faster and momentum builds.

That, in a nutshell, is my system for changing the culture of a health care organization. For a much more in-depth exploration of the Flywheel and its components, please read *Hardwiring Excellence*—but this brief explanation should provide a context in which to consider the all-important role of the physician.

Here's the bottom line: a hospital or medical practice can not live up to its potential without fully engaged physicians, who in the end, can drive the commitment, passion and performance of an organization when they lead by example.

We *all* want to create outstanding places for employees to work, physicians to practice, and patients to receive care. *Practicing Excellence: A Physician's Manual to Exceptional Health Care* is one more beacon illuminating our path to that noble—and achievable— goal.

Quint Studer

A Note from the Author

As I wrote this book, I sought to provide physicians and health care leaders tactical guidance to create exceptional care for patients. Few would disagree that providing exceptional care to patients is the right thing to do, but implementing and executing physician excellence for every patient, every time requires physician engagement, training, and organizational culture change. Changing a culture in health care is about a willingness to commit to clinical and service excellence as a non-negotiable expectation of staff physicians, and to create physician commitment so they lead this effort through example and influence on all who look to them for leadership. This pathway to achieve full physician engagement is the objective of this book.

Physician engagement is ultimately about a willingness of physicians to lead, and a passion to never settle for anything short of exceptional when it comes to taking care of patients. What is it that makes a physician do this and lead efforts to excellence?

Perhaps most foundational to cultivating and navigating physician change is to realize its simplicity. The most important element of change does not lie necessarily in the tools, training, accountability, measurement, incentives, organizational standards, or even the leadership of your institution. True change manifests when values, beliefs, experiences, and convictions fuel a passion to make a difference. Change happens when physicians can step away from the intensity of the day and look at care through the eyes of patients.

Change will occur when the best day we have is the one that is measured by the unmistakable fulfillment that comes to us from patients through our provision of kindness and compassion. Sustained change happens when physicians realize that we can cure sometimes, but we can make a difference with every patient, every time. At the end of the day, the physician change effort will be nurtured and fed by touching the lives of patients and families. The dedication to others is what allows certain physicians to rise above others, lead by example, and make everyone they touch better.

Through clinical failure, I learned the depth of the impact of what we do. A mother of three young children came to my office complaining of back pain. At 37 years old, she was three years out from a bone marrow transplant after ablative chemotherapy for breast cancer (a procedure that is no longer done), and our team of oncologists had followed her closely. Given her history and severity of pain, I ordered a lumbar x-ray. She returned from radiology several minutes later with her films in hand, anxious to see what it was that had kept her up at night for the last few weeks. I placed the films on the viewing board. Her spine and pelvis were riddled with metastatic disease. I turned to her, unable to tell her what I knew. I told her I needed to review the films with the radiologist and I would see her the next day to review the findings. She knew something was wrong. I didn't sleep wondering how to tell a mother and wife that she had a terminal cancer. She returned the next day with her husband, prepared to ask questions that I was ill-equipped to answer. "Is the cancer back?" "Yes," I said, trying to look directly at a young woman who was just told she would die soon. Her face fell into her hands and she began to sob. Her husband wrapped his arms around her desperately trying to hold himself together but quickly gave way to their brutal reality. The next several months were filled with aggressive chemotherapy protocols, intractable pain, nausea, baldness, and amazing spirit to relish every day she had.

The chemo did little to arrest the disease, and she came to the hospital a final time to relieve her pain. We gave her a private room so she could be alone with her family. We met with her for hours discussing her case and the options available. The fact was we had nothing left to offer. I spoke with her husband two to three times every day as he watched his wife die. I watched him kiss her forehead again and again as she drifted away. I consoled and comforted him the best I could. I watched their small children hug their mom and say goodbye knowing that her death was imminent. The family gathered in a conference room as we communicated and anticipated that she would pass at any moment. Her comfort was maintained and she died peacefully with her family at her side.

The husband called me the following day to thank me for being her physician. He thanked me for treating her like family, and helping them get through a treacherous time. His children and his wife were the same age as mine.

I realized on that day the potential of what we do goes far beyond just the medicine. The true impact of medicine is more than the chemotherapy protocol, the radiation treatment, the surgery, the angiography, or the antibiotic. In the face of clinical failure, I learned what medicine can do and I haven't looked back since.

The tools and training in this manual create a roadmap that ultimately leads to the simplicity of physician change. The manual will provide the tools and training for the execution of excellence, but it is the touch and compassion of the human spirit that matter most. As we follow this roadmap, it will allow us to utilize the leadership of engaged, impassioned physicians trained to be the best, and inspired to make a difference.

Stephen C. Beeson, MD

To my beautiful wife, Deanna, and amazing kids, Sydney and Nicholas. Thank you for your love, support, and sacrifices.

To patients everywhere, who deserve nothing but the best.

INTRODUCTION

It is amazing that so much of a medical organization's success or failure rides on the conduct and performance of its physicians, and yet so little time is spent providing physicians the tools and training that are the requisites for this success. The correlation of clinical outcomes and service provided to patients by physicians has become undeniable. Clinical success comes not only from the skill of the treating physician, but, equally important, from our ability to establish communication, partnership, and trust with those who have entrusted their lives in our care.

One could say that the medical marketplace now judges us more by virtue of our ability to communicate than by our ability to diagnose and treat. The combination of technical excellence and premier service has become inseparable, and one without the other is now insufficient. The reason is simple: our patients don't have the ability to assess our clinical talent, and they assume that we can do what we spent a decade or more to learn. Our extraordinary technical abilities have now become an assumption. The principle means we have to manage, market, and convey our talent rides directly on the coattails of our ability to communicate and collaborate with our patients.

So, how does a physician, in the midst of a 25 patient day, 30 phone messages, 40 prescription refill requests, hospital rounds, and "managing" a large clinical practice, do the things that need to be done to foster satisfaction and loyalty amongst the patients we see?

Regardless of your organizational circumstances, the tools physicians use to provide the patients what they deserve and what the marketplace demands do not change. The success of our practice now depends on execution of skills for which we receive little or no training. The tools written in this manual are offered with the intent of providing the physician behaviors that will foster patient satisfaction, but perhaps more importantly, create a workplace built on collaboration, commitment, purpose, and making a difference. The tools in this manual are meant principally for the benefit of the patients we treat, but if you take a careful look at physicians with extraordinary careers, you will often find that they are the physicians who have dedicated themselves to the values, ethics, and conduct that are inherent in the behaviors articulated in this manual. Many will say we best serve ourselves by our dedication to others.

I joined this profession to make a difference in the lives of the patients and families I treat. In health care, nothing short of exceptional should do. If you have this manual in your hands, I know you feel the same way.

CHAPTER 1:
THE CULTURE OF EXCELLENCE

The creation of a Culture of Excellence within a health care organization is a relentless transformational process to become the best place to work, the best place to practice medicine, and the best place to receive care. The creation of a Culture of Excellence is not about slogans, motivational speakers, or market strategies, but rather building and implementing systems that hardwire operations, service, and behaviors that deliver tangible results.

Hardwiring excellence within a health care organization is a comprehensive process requiring:

- An unwavering organizational commitment to excellence
- The creation and development of leaders
- Measurement of organizational progress
- The engagement, support, and leadership of physicians
- The building of a culture around service
- Dedication to employee satisfaction
- Accountability for performance at every level
- Behaviors aligned with the values and mission of the institution
- Clear, continual communication of the organizational progress, mission, and values to every unit
- An environment where the best in the organization are continually recognized and where there is a constitutional intolerance to low performance

1

The patient experience within an organization that has transformed its culture and hardwired its values and behaviors is a patient experience that no longer depends on which staff, which shift, which nurse, which department, or which physician. Premier care simply happens with every patient, every time.

Patients will be acknowledged and greeted as though each of the staff members have been waiting specifically for them. Staff and physicians will make eye contact, smile, and say "hello" to patients and colleagues as they walk the hallways of the facility. Nurses, receptionists, and physicians will introduce themselves and what specific role they play in the care of the patient. Care providers will proudly reveal their experience, expertise, and training to patients to assure the patients that their care is in the hands of experts. Patients will have specific durations of appointments, procedures, and waiting times explained and communicated every time. Staff and physicians

---

The patient experience within an organization that has transformed its culture and hardwired its values and behaviors is a patient experience that no longer depends on which staff, which shift, which nurse, which department, or which physician.

---

will explain everything that will happen with the care of the patients to include what is involved, why it is being done, how long it will take, if it will hurt, and what the next step of care will be. Everyone involved in the care of the patients will make extensive efforts to be sure all the patients' questions are answered. Patients will be taken where they need to go should they lose their way. Staff and physicians will position each other and the organization well to reduce patient anxiety and profile their commitment to be the best. Patient phone calls will be returned in the time frame to which the staff commits.

Patients will be thanked for coming to the facility and entrusting the physicians and nurses in their care. Most importantly, all patients will be treated with kindness, respect, and compassion. Every patient, every time.

The organization becomes known for delivering exceptional care and service to all of its patients at every contact point, from the receptionist, nurse, physician, phlebotomist, physical therapist, x-ray technician, security guard, and volunteer. Prescriptive expectations of conduct become so pervasive that those who don't embrace the commitment of the organization must get better or leave. High-performing staff will interview and select their own peers, and prospective applicants will be chosen based upon prior performance and their match with the culture of the institution. All new employees will have orientation and training supporting established standards of conduct as conditions and expectations of employment. The organization that has implemented a Culture of Excellence then becomes a living, breathing advertisement for itself from the testimony of every patient who walks through the doors. The pride that invariably comes with prescriptive excellence yields tangible results with objective measures. More importantly, the pride that comes from making a difference for patients continues to drive the organization to higher levels of performance and achievement. The

---

The organization that has implemented a Culture of Excellence then becomes a living, breathing advertisement for itself from the testimony of every patient who walks through the doors.

---

better the organization gets, the better the organization becomes, and the more the organization demands of itself.

THE PHYSICIANS' ROLE

The physicians' role is foundational in the creation of operational and service excellence. Physicians are the clinical workplace leaders and will set the tone for how care is to be delivered. How physicians treat patients, staff, and each other will establish the benchmark and standards of conduct for the organization. If the commitment, conduct, and performance of physicians are not aligned with the organizational commitment to excellence, the organization will be unable to rise above the level practiced by the clinical workplace leaders.

Many good physicians can speak exhaustively about sub-optimal practice conditions that prevent them from engaging and committing to the fundamental behaviors that can ultimately get them to where they would like to be. Physicians often wait for the perfect alignment of practice operations before they feel they can provide exceptional care experiences to their patients: "I would have higher patient satisfaction if we had better staff, if the staff had better training, if I had another FTE." "I would have better patient

---

If the commitment, conduct, and performance of physicians are not aligned with the organizational commitment to excellence, the organization will be unable to rise above the level of the perceived clinical workplace leaders.

---

satisfaction if I had more time with my patients, if they weren't so sick, if they weren't from such a high socioeconomic group, if they weren't from such a low socioeconomic group, if I didn't have so many HMO patients, if I had a better payer mix…"

The fact is that the physician who continually stands on the sideline listing reasons for low patient and staff satisfaction, and does not assume personal responsibility for how care is to be delivered, is a physician whose results will never improve. When physicians make

---

Physicians cannot wait for operational excellence to justify their commitment; they need to achieve excellence through influence, example, and leadership.

---

arguments for their own limitations, those limitations will become their own, and can stifle the progress of the organization.

The Culture of Excellence will never come passively into our practice. A Culture of Excellence comes from the leadership of those who have the greatest impact on the conduct of others. Physicians cannot wait for operational excellence to justify their commitment; they need to achieve excellence through influence, example, and leadership.

Physician conduct that drives organizational excellence is founded in how we treat staff, how we treat patients, and how we treat each other. One element is no less important than another. The physician who treats patients with expertise, care, and compassion, but micromanages and bullies his staff will undermine the clinical team's ability to deliver that same level of care and service. Our staff will treat our patients just like we treat them.

How physicians treat each other within a medical group remains a principle predictor of the physician workplace experience, and will cultivate an organization's performance culture. Teamwork amid physicians supports the overarching group mission over individual agendas. Collegiality allows physicians to cover each other for illnesses, family deaths, and new babies, and fosters partnership and loyalty to the group and its mission.

The relationship between physicians and administrative leadership can have a significant impact on the effectiveness of your administrative team to drive institutional results. In fact, without the visibility of physician involvement, the administrative team's ability to implement and hardwire frontline staff behaviors is limited. Leadership can train all they want, but if your staff doesn't see behaviors modeled by leaders, most of all physicians, behavioral change is not sustainable within your organization.

PHYSICIAN CHANGE

In the end, the cultural transformation of a medical organization is one that is founded on leaders' ability to drive and sustain change. Historically, physicians have not been on the forefront of change when it comes to practice operations and how care is delivered to patients. It is important to understand the complexity of factors that influence physician change, since this is the pathway that one must navigate to create and sustain physician and organizational excellence.

Different physicians begin to change for different reasons. Some will make an effort for change with a simple reminder of the impact they can have by doing things differently. Others will continue to stand in protest despite a compelling body of evidence that service excellence drives clinical and practice success. Successful and thorough physician engagement is about understanding physicians and speaking to the issues and principles that inspire, motivate, incentivize, influence, and push a physician's commitment to a change effort.

The principal drivers for physician behavioral change include the following:

Knowledge. When physicians learn the prospective benefit of a tactical behavior to improve an outcome measure compared to what has been done before, physicians become more amenable to change.

Communicating the "evidence for service" is fundamental to a physician's understanding of the benefit and need for change.

Training. Providing prescriptive behavioral training to physicians is foundational to performance improvement. Physicians must be taught the behaviors that work to drive the patient experience and enhance staff performance. Providing behavioral training to physicians can influence behavior, but training efforts must be recurrent. A single didactic exposure is not enough to sustain long-term change.

Data Feedback. Feedback of performance information in regards to patient satisfaction or quality measures to physicians can potentially be a powerful agent of change. Optimal motivation for change will occur when the data is presented in a systematic, comparative fashion. How physicians compare to colleagues in a national comparative database will often stir a physician's effort to improve. Profiled results have the greatest impact when data is transparent to colleagues.

Colleague Influence. The perception, opinion, and attitudes of respected physician colleagues can impact a physician's willingness to change clinical practice patterns, conduct, and behaviors. What your respected physician leaders say "off the record" about the mission of your group will have a heavy influence on the perceived worthiness of organizational efforts. Physicians of power in your organization must be aligned with the objectives of the institution to harness support and buy-in amongst colleagues.

Organizational Expectations. The expectations articulated by the organization can influence what physicians will do. When expectations are not well communicated or profiled, physicians are less likely to conform to the "code of conduct" of the organization. When clear expectations are used for orientation and training, and standards are repeatedly voiced by leaders within the organization, a sense of importance is created and physician behavioral adherence becomes more likely.

Incentives. Monetary incentives can change physician behaviors in regards to clinical measures[1] and productivity,[2] but the impact on non-clinical performance and behavior is less clear. Interviews of practicing physicians report that financial incentives did not substantially affect their own behavior, but interviews of medical group leaders revealed a sense that financial incentives do impact physician behaviors.[3] Financial incentives seem to have some impact on what physicians do, and behavior change is likely related to the size of "at risk" monies, with 10-15 percent of income at risk for incentivized performance measures enough to change behaviors in most groups.[4]

Patient Expectations. Patient "demand" can have a major influence on what physicians do. Physicians often practice with the reality that the patients have researched and read about their symptoms or disease, and come to seek the physician's opinion on what they have learned. Additionally, patients expect to partner with physicians in their care and are no longer passive recipients of our opinion and recommendations.

Recognition. Recognition for physicians by patients, colleagues, or leadership for doing something well increases the likelihood that those behaviors will continue.

Emotional Persuasion. The most successful efforts of behavioral change speak to the emotional response to elicited change.[5] Does a behavioral change create an emotional response that will reinforce and nourish the change effort? This concept is the basis for sustained physician behavioral change perhaps above all else. The emotional persuasion for physicians is a personal, tangible experience that can change attitudes, values, and behaviors in a sustainable way. If providing exceptional care to patients creates fulfillment and joy in what we do, this may be the most important change element of all.

The pathway to an organizational Culture of Excellence is understanding what it is that inspires change, and what creates a willingness to step out of patterns of behaviors that have been engrained for decades. Creating tactics for true physician and organizational transformation requires engagement of not singular efforts, but a broad multi-front approach, running concurrently. All of the known drivers and motivators for physician change must be organizationally deployed to assure the best chance for physician behavioral change. The tools and tactics communicated in this manual are fundamentally about transforming what physicians do and will provide prescriptive guidance to full physician engagement.

CHAPTER 2:

THE CASE FOR SERVICE

Service to patients goes far beyond common courtesies and friendliness. Service to patients is about collaboration, establishing trust, clear communication, empathy, listening, and conducting ourselves in a way that reflects that improving patients' comfort and outcome is the most important thing we do. Compelling evidence has shown that patients make their health care decisions based on the service provided by physicians. According to a Harris Poll published in the *Wall Street Journal* in September 2004:

"People place more importance on doctors' interpersonal skills than their medical judgment or experience, and doctors' failings in these areas are the overwhelming factor that drives patients to switch doctors."

No one would question the fact that the service physicians provide to patients correlates strongly with patient satisfaction. But one could make equally convincing arguments that service provided to patients by physicians can increase economic returns, reduce malpractice risk, improve patient adherence to treatment recommendations, improve clinical outcomes, reduce physician burnout, improve staff satisfaction and retention, and can help create the kinds of patients that physicians enjoy caring for.

Recently, I saw a patient who had returned from a consultation I had arranged. The consultant was a physician who was well known, respected, and clinically talented. When the patient sat in my office, I asked how his appointment went. He said to me, "I'm not sure." "What do you mean?" I asked. "Well, he really didn't say much in regards to the issue that I thought I was seeing him for. He gave me a prescription, with no explanation as to what it was for or why I was to take it, how long I was supposed to be on it, and what the side effects were." The patient continued to explain, clearly rekindling the irritation and annoyance that was created from the visit. "Then he left before I had a chance to ask him a single question. I finally found his nurse to ask a few questions about the medication. She told me that he had moved on to the next patient and if I had any questions I could call back later."

The patient didn't call the physician to follow up on the visit, nor did the patient fill the prescription. The value of the visit and the prospective clinical benefit was zero as a result of poor service and communication. Service to patients is about using communication and collaborative techniques to create clinical influence and better outcomes for patients.

THE CASE FOR SERVICE—PATIENT COMPLIANCE

Physicians often will assess themselves and colleagues by their ability to diagnose and treat disease. That is a fair benchmark because that is our role and that is what we are trained to do. What is critical to understand, though, is that our ability to treat patients effectively will be predicted by our ability to get the patients to understand and do what we ask them. Our ability to provide and impart care is predicted by a number of factors. Clear communication provided by a trusted physician will predict patient compliance and satisfaction with care. Satisfied patients are more likely to comply with treatment, more likely to assume an active role in their care, and to continue medical care with their current physician, when other choices are available. [6 7 8]

Satisfied patients are more likely to comply with treatment, more likely to assume an active role in their care, and to continue medical care with their current physician.

According to the Office of the Inspector General, noncompliance with medications results in 125,000 deaths each year from cardiovascular disease alone. In other studies, it has been estimated that noncompliance is responsible for 10-25 percent of all hospital and nursing home admissions.[9 10] In studies of patient behavior, only about half of patients who leave a physician's office with a prescription take the drug as directed.[11] Children taking antibiotics had even lower compliance rates. Nearly 60 percent of children stopped treatment by the third day of a known streptococcal throat infection, and 82 percent stopped treatment by the ninth day.[12] It is estimated that only 30-40 percent of those who are prescribed statin therapy comply at one year of treatment, followed by ongoing gradual decline thereafter.[13] In fact, poor compliance has been reported as the most common cause of nonresponse to medications.[14]

These disturbing findings have driven many experts to conclude that patient noncompliance is one of the most important problems in health care today. The consistent predictors of patient compliance are the trust, collaboration, and communication that patients have with their physicians.

Physicians' communication skills can heavily influence patient compliance and will impact clinical outcomes. For example, a study of emergency room physician interactions demonstrated that establishing rapport with patients shows a relationship to patient compliance with emergency room directions.[15] In another study, women whose physicians discussed mammography with some or a great deal of enthusiasm were four and a half times more likely to report having a mammogram compared to women whose physician had little or no enthusiasm.[16] Additionally, when physicians provide information to patients regarding their diagnosis and treatment that allows the patients to understand the importance of self-management in diabetes, self-management practices were actually followed.[17] Studies also have demonstrated that when a physician is approachable, gives serious consideration to the patient's concerns, and communicates well, better patient compliance is likely.[18]

How is it that in the United States we spend over $200 billion per year on prescription medications, and billions more on research and development of pharmaceuticals, but physicians often fail to spend the two critical minutes to provide the information and communication to patients that is the necessity of compliance?

Our ability to be clinically effective and to drive outcomes with proposed treatment is clearly dependent on our ability to communicate and partner with patients. Writing a prescription and darting out of the exam room, without providing information and a query of patient understanding, will, more times than not, result in noncompliance with a treatment regimen. The best treatment plan in the world does not matter if the patient doesn't follow it.

THE CASE FOR SERVICE—GROWTH, MARKET SHARE, AND LOYALTY

Many health care organizations would hit growth objectives if they could simply stop losing the patients they currently have. The cost of acquiring a new patient is five to seven times greater than retaining current ones.[19] Additionally, loyal patients are the most vocal in telling others about the care and service they received, are more tolerant of minor office-related problems that can arise, and have the greatest impact on revenue through repeat visits and referrals. The fundamental question that arises is: *What is it that drives the patients' health care decision making?* What will make them come to a facility in the first place, and what is it that makes them stay when other options are available?

The answers to these marketplace queries are nestled directly on the shoulders of the patient experience with a health care organization, and more specifically with the physician providing their care. Core service does not generate loyalty. Exceeding expectations with exceptional service keeps patients coming back. It has been shown that patients who are extremely satisfied with the care and services provided by their physician are willing to make financial sacrifices and endure inconvenience to stay in their care. The requisite for this loyalty is something special about the service provided to patients that occurs with every encounter. If patients are merely "satisfied," they can and will go elsewhere should circumstances for change arise. Communication, attitude, respect, reliability, empathy, and kindness are physician and organizational traits that distinguish a practice that creates loyalty amongst the patients they treat. Nearly 70 percent of all health care choices are made by word of mouth.[20] What patients say to their friends, family, and colleagues about a medical group and its physicians can determine the competitiveness and long-term viability of an organization. It is the difference between good and great that earns patients for a lifetime, and it is the chasm that many physicians and organizations fail to cross.

"The gulf between satisfied and completely satisfied customers can swallow a business."

Harvard Business Review, December 1995

THE CASE FOR SERVICE—MALPRACTICE RISK

Physician conduct and communication, and not necessarily untoward clinical outcomes, appear to be the principle predictors of malpractice risk. In fact, recent evidence suggests the surprising realization that the initiation of lawsuits bears no direct relationship to the severity of patient harm. For example, although 1 percent of hospitalized patients develop a significant injury related to negligence, less than 3 percent of those decide to sue the physicians providing their care. Thus, the great majority of injured patients do not initiate lawsuits.[21] What is it that differentiates the 3 percent of harmed patients who sue from the 97 percent of harmed patients who do not? In one recent review of malpractice depositions, 71 percent of all claims were related to a breakdown in physician/patient communication.[22]

Physician conduct and communication, and not necessarily untoward clinical outcomes, appear to be the principle predictors of malpractice risk.

In studies evaluating patient satisfaction and malpractice risk, it was found that a relatively small number of physicians generate a disproportionate number of complaints from patients and malpractice lawsuits. In a survey conducted of inpatients over a three-year period, it was found that physicians in the lowest 33rd percentile for patient satisfaction had a 110 percent increase in malpractice risk and a 140 percent increase in complaints compared to those physicians in the upper 33rd percentile.[23] Another study reported that within a variety of specialties, 3 to 8 percent of physicians were responsible for 75 to 85 percent of all payments for awards and settlements, with surgeons with two or more malpractice claims having nearly six times as many complaints as their colleagues with no lawsuits.[24] Unsolicited patient complaints are undeniably identifiers for malpractice suit risk.[25]

In obstetrical practices, patients seeing physicians with a high number of malpractice claims were significantly more likely to complain that they felt rushed, never received explanations for tests, and were often ignored.[26]

In primary care, a study was performed looking at communication styles of "no-claim" physicians with no prior lawsuits, vs. "claims" physicians with more than one prior claim. In comparison, no-claim physicians spent more time educating patients about what to expect next and the flow of the visit. They laughed and used humor more, and spent more time partnering with patients and soliciting their understanding. On average, the no-claim physician spent two to three minutes more per patient visit compared to the claims physician.[27]

The evidence for effective and collaborative communication between physician and patient reducing malpractice risk is very strong and has been duplicated in numerous studies. The next logical question that arises is: *Can physicians learn to communicate more effectively with patients, or is it simply inherent?* Are some physicians just doomed to poor performance and malpractice risk?

Significant data exist that suggest physicians can improve communication skills, and with these improved skills, can yield tangible improvements in patient satisfaction, clinical outcomes, and malpractice exposure risk. In fact, physician training has demonstrated that physician conduct and communication can change significantly, and physicians were able to do this without having to spend any more time with patients.[28]

Numerous studies have made consistent conclusions regarding the most protective strategies against malpractice claims. Physician service excellence, delivered through communication, collaboration, respect, and trust with patients, correlates highly with significant reductions of lawsuit probability.[29]

THE CASE FOR SERVICE—PHYSICIAN RELATIONSHIPS TO STAFF

In terms of the performance of the organization, how physicians treat their staff may be as important as what physicians do for patients. The conduct of physicians can have a powerful impact on staff satisfaction and the staff workplace experience and will influence staff performance. Staff will act on the basis of their workplace perception. They will gripe, complain, and use poor judgment with patients if the work they do is habitually unnoticed, if they feel their contribution has no purpose, if they are not trained and empowered to do their jobs, or if they don't have the tools and equipment to do their work effectively.

A healthy physician-nurse relationship is not just a nice thing to have; it is a competitive advantage driving clinical outcomes, patient safety, and staff retention. Interviews of nurses demonstrate that when physicians intimidate and behave disruptively, clinical care is impacted.[30] Ninety-two percent of hospital-based nursing staff have witnessed disruptive physician behaviors and report a compromise in communication, collaboration, and information transfer. Nurses also reported disruptive physicians increase frustration, stress, and the quality of workplace relationships. When respectful, collaborative physician-nurse communication is in place, and nurses are encouraged to speak-up in the face of patient danger, errors are reduced and care for patients improves.

Patient satisfaction improves when each physician-nurse team has a clear, shared vision of how patients will be treated that is in alignment with the service culture. When physicians communicate a commitment to service excellence to staff and lead by example, their behavior can be a powerful reinforcer to service training underway within an organization. Example is not the main way to influence others; it is the only way.

Example is not the main way of influencing others;
it is the only way.

One of the best physicians I know, with whom I would entrust the care of my own family, and whose patient satisfaction ranks him amongst the best in the country, has a difficult time keeping nurses. He has been described as a micromanager, constantly hovering over his nurses, and having a hand in every phone call and every decision throughout the workday. Nurses become frustrated and resentful that they are unable to do the job they were trained to do. This constant frustration from nurses invariably impacts their disposition and loyalty to the organization, the physician, and even to the patients. Organizational performance is compromised by the interaction and relationship of the physician to his staff. Despite being staffed with "excellent" physicians, the office site is plagued by high turnover, frustration, and low patient satisfaction. Until the issue was addressed, this physician had no idea the ripple effect his style was having on his support staff.

Just as negative physician behavior can undermine workplace performance, it is equally clear that positive physician behavior and attitude can foster staff retention, loyalty, and satisfaction while promoting behaviors in alignment with the mission of your group. Simple strategies like thanking your nurses at the end of the day for the work they do creates the recognition environment that improves staff loyalty. Physicians who identify and communicate the good work of staff and "manage up" others will reproduce recognized and praised behaviors.

---

*Never underestimate how important just a few moments spent
focused on the personal well-being of those around you can be to
make your staff feel valued, appreciated, and a part of the team.*

The physician's role in workplace operations and performance is
critical. Physicians are in a leadership position and will influence the
perception, attitudes, and behaviors of others. A vested physician
committed to reward and recognition, who clearly articulates
expectations, who gets to know and takes care of staff, and models
the behaviors consistent with their organizational mission, will create
a high-performing unit. When receptionists, nurses, and ancillary
staff are in proximity to impassioned physicians who demand
excellence of themselves, they too become better. It's not about
waiting for operational excellence to come to you; it's about creating
operational and service excellence yourself through leadership,
influence, and example.

THE CASE FOR SERVICE—PHYSICIAN RELATIONSHIPS TO COLLEAGUES

How physicians within your organization treat each other may
be the least referenced, but most important predictor of physician
satisfaction. Traditionally, extrinsic operational elements, such as
workload, physician autonomy, and income, have been the strongest
perceived correlates to physician satisfaction. More recent studies,
however, look deeper into what it is that predicts the environment in
which a physician will thrive professionally and grow personally.

The important determinant of the fulfillment of a physician's day
is not necessarily the number of patients we evaluate and treat, the
phone calls that we return to patients, or the time we are able to

finish work and go home to see our families. The quality of the work experience often will lie in the collaborative environment in which we do our work. Physician groups flourish when physicians simply get along with each other and are willing to create cooperation and consensus on the fundamental operations of the group. Physician groups thrive when there are systematic efforts to share clinical knowledge and expertise where the skills and talents of each physician are best utilized for the collective good. Physician groups thrive when physicians position each other well in the eyes of patients and staff, and where differences are clarified respectfully and openly for the good of patient care. Physician groups thrive when the needs of the patient, and the prevailing mission and culture of the organization, supercede the personal agenda of any single physician.

The service that physicians provide to each other is a critical component in the fabric of the physician day-to-day experience. A physician who has colleagues who are willing to help each other is highly protective against physician dissatisfaction, frustration, and burnout. Collegiality and collaboration amongst physicians is a predictor of organizational success and will drive physician satisfaction, performance, and willingness to embrace organizational values.

A physician who has colleagues who are willing to help each other is highly protective against physician dissatisfaction, frustration, and burnout.

Physician service to patients will drive patient satisfaction, compliance, and clinical outcomes. Physician service to staff will create committed, loyal, and high-performing staff willing to "go to battle" with you any day of the week. Physician service to physician colleagues, though, may be the most important investment we make to create a group of physicians who support each other, help each other, defend each other, and laugh together in what can be a physically, intellectually, and emotionally exhausting profession. Physicians' serving each other never will be measured on any outcome matrix; however, it is crucial to sustain the health, commitment, sanity, vigor, and spirit of your physicians to do the work of caring for others. You will find that physician camaraderie, collaboration, and friendship lie under the hood of the medical groups in this country who have established distinguished histories of being the best. Never underestimate their importance.

Key Learning Points—The Case for Service

1. Service provided to patients can be more important than clinical experience in determining health care choices for patients today.

2. Noncompliance remains a major public health problem and can be effectively improved through communication and collaboration with patients on treatment plans.

3. Loyal patients are greater revenue producers than acquiring new patients.

4. Patient loyalty is determined not by "core services," but by receiving a service that was beyond what was expected.

5. Malpractice risk is predicted by communication abilities of physicians:

    a. Complaints predict malpractice risk.

    b. Higher patient satisfaction reduces malpractice risk.

    c. Communication breakdown is the most common reason cited for filing claims.

6. Physicians can improve staff morale, performance, and retention through:

    a. Investing in relationships.

    b. Clear, constructive, respectful communication.

    c. Specific reward and recognition.

    d. Modeling behaviors consistent with the organizational mission.

7. Physicians can improve physician satisfaction through:

    a. Collegiality and respect amongst physicians.

    b. A willingness to help colleagues.

    c. A common mission, to which each physician upholds.

    d. Positioning each other well to patients (managing up).

CHAPTER 3:
PHYSICIAN SERVICE EXCELLENCE TOOLS

It is becoming progressively clear what is important to patients when they see a physician. While every patient is different, tremendous commonalities exist in creating the collaboration, trust, partnership, and loyalty that every patient and physician desires. The literature is so overwhelming in terms of the impact of service and communication on clinical outcomes, malpractice risk, loyalty, growth, patient satisfaction, and organizational success, that it really is no longer up for debate. Once we concede that service excellence is foundational to our success as physicians and the groups we work with, the question is no longer a matter of if, but a matter of how and when we will deploy the tools that will get results. Medical groups simply cannot compete in this current medical marketplace without engaging the tools that work to drive the patient experience.

An organization simply cannot compete in this current medical marketplace without engaging the tools that work to drive the patient experience.

This chapter is the "how-to" portion of this manual, providing prescriptive, evidence-based guidance to every element of the patient encounter, including:

- Creating the first impression with patients
- What you need to know before entering the exam room
- Techniques in history taking
- The physician exam
- Providing patient information
- Patient partnership and collaboration
- Positioning your colleagues well (managing up)
- Patient follow-up
- Effective appointment closure

These tools, used properly, will take no more time than what you spend currently, and will land you and your group amongst the best in the nation in the eyes of patients. It is not a question of whether the tools work, but a question of who will commit to using them for every patient, every time.

THE FIRST IMPRESSION

Human behavior dictates that in every new situation, a first impression is created. It is thought that judgment can be passed within the first several seconds of an interaction, and it is known that the best of first impressions creates a captive and engaged encounter, and a poor first impression is just plain difficult to recover from. In order for a physician to convey kindness, compassion, intelligence, confidence, and commitment to the well-being of a new patient, the first impression we create is critical. The following are fundamental components to creating a positive first impression with patients.

In order for a physician to convey kindness, compassion, intelligence,
confidence, and commitment to the well-being of a new patient,
the first impression we create is critical.

1. Knock on the door before entering.
- A common courtesy and a conveyance of your respect for their privacy and apprehension.
- Pause for two seconds prior to room entry, thus preparing the patient for your entrance.

Recently, in an ongoing effort to keep my patients informed, I poked my head in the room of a waiting patient to let her know how long I would be. This poor young woman was entirely naked standing in the middle of the exam room. I now knock for everyone, every time.

2. Smile, introduce yourself, and shake the patient's hand. Be sure to acknowledge and introduce yourself to others who may have accompanied the patient. Anyone who enters an exam room with a patient is personally close and important to that patient.
- Friendliness of a physician will improve patient comfort and satisfaction with you,[31] and the ability to have the honest, forthright relationship that is clinically effective.
- A smile places the patient at ease, the first step in creating confidence and comfort in the eyes of patients.
- A smile conveys that we enjoy what we do; it begins building trust and reduces patient anxiety.
- Don't look preoccupied and irritated, even if you are. Develop the ability to leave your issues outside.

3. Sit and maintain eye contact. This may be the most important biomechanical component of your visit.

- When physicians sit during the course of the interview, it will significantly increase the patients' perception of time spent with them compared to those who stand, without actually spending any more time. Consider this a must-have for every patient interview.
- Face the patient if possible. Physicians' facing more than 45 degrees away from the patient has a negative correlation to the patient's perception of the encounter.[32]

4. Use consistent opening comments. Create a list of introductory comments that you can use for new and established patients that will establish the tone of the visit in a way that is most effective and constructive for the patient and you. **A non-medical dialogue is effective in reinforcing the strong first impression you have created and places the patient at ease.** What you say to new and established patients is distinctly different. Depending on the patient and the situation, the following is a demonstration of what can be said to new patients:

OPENING DIALOGUE WITH NEW PATIENTS (PRIMARY CARE):

> *"Hi, I'm Dr. Beeson. Nice to meet you. Have a seat; make yourself comfortable. Well, I see you are a new patient here. Thank you for coming in and welcome to the Sharp Rees-Stealy Medical Group. Did everything go smoothly in terms of your registration and check-in? Did my staff treat you well? Excellent. I know how fun it can be to see your new physician for the first time (smile at the patient), so I would like to make this as comfortable and easy as we can for you. Tell me a little about yourself."*

This new patient introduction is natural, simple, and places the patient at ease in an inviting, friendly exchange that is the prerequisite for a meaningful clinical dialogue. Use humor when you can. Laughter makes a notable, positive impact on patients[33] and conveys unhurriedness and approachability. Sometimes you will need to prompt nervous or reserved patients to tell you if they work in the area, what they do for a living, do they have family, do they have children, or whatever seems appropriate. Most patients enjoy and are most comfortable talking about themselves. The most important feature in this initial contact is that you create an environment that instills comfort for the patients.

Following the opening dialogue, tell patients about your training, education, and experience. Take a moment to communicate with patients your personal approach and philosophy toward patient care. Patients must believe they are beginning a relationship with a physician who is accessible, receptive, listens, and acts in a way that makes them confident that you care about them and they are in expert hands. As with all behaviors that drive the patient experience, it is of greatest importance that you commit to performing them without exception. Every patient, every time.

OPENING DIALOGUE WITH ESTABLISHED PATIENTS (PRIMARY CARE):

> *"Hi, Bob…nice to see you again. Thank you for waiting…I know I am running a few minutes behind this morning. Sit down and make yourself comfortable. So, how's life been treating you these days?"*

Even for patients you have known for years, a smooth, simple, and friendly greeting lays the foundation for a fruitful clinical encounter. If you are running more than 15 minutes past the scheduled time, thank them for waiting. Even with operational efficiency, offices will, at times, if not most times, run behind. If you are more than 30 minutes behind, you will need to proactively acknowledge your delay as you enter the exam room.

Consider the following when arriving excessively late:

"I know you were excited about spending all morning with us in our reception area [laughter]…thank you for waiting. We had some complicated cases this morning but I know it can be frustrating to have to wait so long…nice to see you. So, how has life been treating you these days?"

You will find that this introductory dialogue is almost invariably followed by a palpable recognition of your efforts by even the most irritated patients.

The introductory question of "How has life been treating you?" is a friendly, non-medical query on how they are doing in general. Ideally, for established patients, asking a specific question based upon something you know of them from your history together is a very enriching experience for the patient. Small notes reminding you that Margaret Jones's son is the drum major for the local high school band would create that query opportunity.

The decision to use the patient's first name or title is a personal one for you and the patient. There is no right answer to this question, but many physicians find that with a shared history together over time, using a patient's first name is very natural and helps to reinforce the personal connection between the patient and physician.

These tools to create a first impression and begin an effective clinical encounter convey the most important issue for patients, which is *does this physician and the health care team care about me?* Creating this strong first impression is a prerequisite to all of the important work that we do that follows.

Key Learning Points—First Impressions

1. A good first impression can create a captive, engaged encounter; a bad first impression is difficult to recover from.
2. Knock, then pause two seconds prior to entry.
3. Smile, shake hands, and introduce yourself to the patient and everyone in the room.
4. Sit and sustain eye contact.
5. LOOK AS THOUGH YOU ENJOY WHAT YOU DO!
6. Use a consistent opening dialogue for established and new patients that creates comfort and approachability with you.
7. Tell patients about your training, your experience, and your personal approach to patient care.

EXAM ROOM PREPAREDNESS

The clinical knowledge you have of the patient upon entering the patient exam room will drive the efficiency of clinical care, and can instill or rattle confidence in you as the treating physician. Prior to entering the exam room, review the chart to know of any interval medical events including specialty consultations, surgeries, urgent care or emergency room visits, or follow-up visits with any other physicians. Review the chart to know exactly what you did last for the patient, even if it is not why the patient is coming in today. It is all too common, and distressing to patients, to see their physicians habitually blind-sided by simply not taking the time to review important clinical events clearly available in the medical record.

What you know when you enter the patient exam room will drive the efficiency of clinical care, and can instill or rattle confidence in you as the treating physician.

A patient, who is a close friend of mine, recently described his case to me. He went to see his primary care physician, who has been seeing him every six months or so for the last four years. With every visit, it seemed to the patient that the physician was starting from square one with little recollection of what was done previously. My friend reported that the physician would actually say, "Now, what were we doing again?" My friend would then prompt the physician to remind him that they had increased the dose of his lisinopril and added a low dose diuretic to improve blood pressure control. The physician would ask if he had ordered any labs on him in the last six months. Again, the patient would inform the "treating" physician that no labs were done, and he was not aware of any labs being ordered in the last six months. All the while during this repetitive, ceremonious "I have no idea what I am doing" dialogue with the patient, the physician would be looking frantically through the chart trying to find the answers to the questions that the patient was now providing.

My friend finally left this practice to find a physician with whom he could have confidence and assurance that he was in competent hands.

When medical care becomes more complicated, involving multiple physicians, the task of creating the perception of awareness and knowledge of all that is going on with your patients becomes more demanding and important. The primary care physicians who are judged by patients to be the best are the ones who always seem to know what is going on with their patients, and they deploy specific techniques that create this perception.

When physicians take one to two minutes to make themselves aware of interval events with their patients, this time will be made up in the ability to resume just where they left off, without having to backtrack and backpedal to find out what has been done last.

Let's look at how this is applied in the patient exam room. Let's say it has been three months since your last visit with a patient who you see for glucose intolerance with central obesity and mild hypertension. Three months ago you placed the patient on a low dose ACE inhibitor, sent him to a nutritionist, and reviewed the necessity of diet, exercise, and weight loss to reduce his probability of transitioning to type 2 diabetes. You counseled the patient and collectively agreed that a 10 percent weight loss and 30 minutes per day of cardiovascular exercise was going to be a six-month goal. When the patient comes in for follow-up, you are able to specifically address the issues and goals that you had collaborated on during the last visit. The dialogue could go something like this:

"Last time you were here, we started you on the blood pressure medication lotensin. Tell me how that is going so far." After the patient tells you any interval concerns or questions, you specifically address what your goals were on the last visit and how things are coming along from the patient's perspective. "I see that you saw the nutritionist that we talked about last visit; tell me how that went for you."

If a patient has an unexpected, unplanned medical event where you were not the treating physician, a brief reference to that event is very powerful in creating the perception that you are "all over it" and you know everything happening with your patient. If your patient was seen in urgent care a month prior for a sinus infection, in the midst of the visit you should say, "I reviewed the records from urgent care. How are your sinuses doing?" The patient will be pleased with your working awareness of his or her care and treatments, even if they are not directly provided by you.

Labs and diagnostic test results are also important to review before you enter the exam room. When patients come in for follow-up on a diagnostic test or laboratory, they will want to know the results. If you have a generalized unawareness of what has happened with your patients and the results of the tests you had ordered for them, they will take that to mean that you either don't care, or that you are overextended and too busy to take personal care of the things that are so important to them.

Information management is becoming so effective that most of us have easy electronic access to every element of care for all of our patients, all of the time. Leverage this technology and share it with patients in the exam room to show them what you have available at your fingertips. Patients who feel they are in good hands with someone who is providing personally attentive care, backed by information technology, drives confidence and loyalty to physicians. Physicians who don't invest the time to make themselves aware of interval medical events and communicate information that is easily available will lose a valuable opportunity to establish trust.

Clinical awareness of your patients should be considered to be a service must-have for physicians. Exam room preparedness, like other service tools for physicians, drives not only the patient experience and opinion of you, but creates the foundation of credibility and personalized care that allow for clinical effectiveness, improved compliance, and better clinical outcomes.

Key Learning Points—Exam Room Preparedness

1. What you know and don't know when you enter the exam room creates or undermines the confidence patients will have in you.
2. Review interval events, consults, and what you did last prior to entering the exam room.
3. Specifically reference your "plan" that was established during the prior visit.
4. Communicate your awareness of interval medical events.
5. Leverage the information available to convey you are attentive and aware of every element of their care.

TECHNIQUES IN HISTORY TAKING

Nearly 90 percent of clinical information used in making a diagnosis is obtained from the skillfully collected history. It is the cornerstone of the medical visit. The fundamental question that we must address as physicians is...*Are we going to conduct the interview on our terms, or are we going to conduct the interview on the patient's terms?* The correct answer to this question is symbolic of a paradigm shift in medical care. Health care today will now be provided as patient-centered care, beginning with the patient-centered interview.

The patient-centered interview is an interview approach that utilizes specific techniques to create collaboration and partnership between the patient and physician. This interview technique allows the patient's principle concerns and questions to drive the visit agenda. Instinctively, some physicians grow nervous when there is discussion of "patient-centered initiatives," concerned that patient-centered care may come at the sacrifice of what we need in terms of time and information. In reality, the patient-centered interview does not take any more time and will create higher patient satisfaction and improved compliance and will derive a clearer clinical picture.

Here are techniques that will lay the foundation for the patient-centered interview:

1. **Allow the patient's major health concerns and questions to drive the agenda of the visit.**

   The "list" generated by this query will drive the encounter. The best approach is to have the nurse perform this function while the patient is in the exam room.

   The initial visit would go something like this:

   "Hi, Mrs. Jones, I'm Nancy. It's nice to see you. I am Dr. Smith's nurse. Dr. Smith and I have worked together for over five years, and you're going to love him...he is the best. **One thing we want to be sure to do during your visit today is to make sure your questions and concerns are addressed and taken care of. Tell me about what you would like to review with Dr. Smith today.**

"Excellent, thank you. I will get your chart ready for Dr. Smith and give him your major questions and concerns. He will be in to see you in about 10 minutes. We are running a few minutes behind. Is there anything I can get to keep you comfortable while you wait?"

This nursing query of the patient concerns is a modified version of the traditional chief complaint. The patient agenda will serve as the visit outline. Physicians will sometimes need to add elements to be sure routine health maintenance and follow-up issues are followed appropriately. An example of a written patient agenda is included for your reference in Chapter 11, Best Practices.

2. Let the patient speak without interruption.

With the patient agenda as a guide, take your history and let the patient speak. The average physician will interrupt a patient after approximately 17 seconds during the opening description of the principle patient concern.[34] Patients perceive interruption by physicians to mean that we don't listen. Listening without interruption can save clinical encounter time by avoiding the doorknob issues that physicians dread.

3. Use continuers.

Staring blankly at patients while they provide you the uninterrupted history provides limited value. Your quietness must convey interest. Continued eye contact, leaning forward, or a periodic head nod work to convey your attentiveness and interest.[35] Using terms like, "Go on," "continue," or "I'm listening" can create connection while the patient provides the clinical story.

4. Paraphrase the patient's history.

Every patient will tell their clinical story in their own words. Sometimes it is a clear, concise timeline that you can write verbatim; other times it is a convoluted mess that needs clarification and guidance. In either case, an important tool for us is to listen carefully to what they are saying. When they are finished, repeat the story back to them, in your words.

Experienced physicians can often summarize a patient history usually with three to four tactical sentences. This conveys two critical things to patients. First, you are listening to what they are saying. Second, you are concerned about getting their clinical history right.

In order for us to be clinically effective and to drive compliance with medications that they may not want to take, and treatments that they may not want to undergo, patients must know that their voice has been heard. Paraphrasing has been demonstrated to be one of the most effective medical interview techniques that will accomplish this task. These tools will lay the foundation and open the door for receptiveness to medical treatments that will follow.

5. **Take control when the patient history loses direction.**
All of us experience this daily: the patient who rambles. The majority of tangential patients who seem to tell you far more insignificant detail than you would ever need or use have a legitimate reason for coming to see you.

Establishing a clear patient agenda and referencing the agenda as a guide for the visit can offset the frequency of this occurrence. Despite preventative efforts, the clinical history can still lose its direction. If after giving the patient at least two minutes of uninterrupted opportunity to tell his or her story, and there is no hope in sight for medically meaningful information, we suggest you take control. Tell the patient, "Clearly there are a lot of things going on right now for you. Tell me what it is that is bothering you most." Or you can ask, "What is it that you are most worried about?"

You will be surprised at how this technique can crystallize this avalanche of complaints, to a clearly articulated worry or concern. Physicians will often use this technique when a patient has a long-standing, chronic problem but somehow had to be seen "today" for this issue, or when the patient's degree of worry seems to be disproportionate to the patient's physical findings.

6. Express empathy.

The ability of physicians to understand and convey the impact of disease and pain on patients is powerful. Despite this fact, physicians rarely express empathy to patients during the course of a typically intense daily physician schedule. It's not that physicians don't feel empathy; it's that we are not in the habit of expressing empathy to patients.

When a single mother of three comes to you with a lumbar strain, unable to move after trying to lift her four-year-old the day before, the physician comment of "I am sure this must be very tough for you" can have a tremendous impact on the value of the visit in the eyes of the patient. You care, and you are concerned about finding the best approach to restore her function and relieve her pain. In fact, physicians' utilization of keywords such as "care" and "comfort" when communicating with patients has a powerful impact on patients' judgment of physicians. The intellectual appreciation of the patient's condition will improve the patient's perception of care.[36] Patient-perceived physician empathy influences patient satisfaction through enhanced perceived expertise, information exchange, interpersonal trust, and partnership.[37] **Tactical and honest expression of empathy by physicians supports the most important predictor of patient satisfaction, which is:** *Did the physician care about me?*

Recognizing when to express empathy simply takes common sense and a caring spirit. Generally, women are more responsive to empathy than men. When a 25-year-old male comes in with a shoulder bursitis after pitching six innings in his adult Tuesday night baseball league, he wants timely intervention, and may not need or respond to empathy.

Key Learning Points—History Taking

1. Ask patients about their concerns and worries to establish the agenda for the visit.
2. Allow patients to speak without interruption (up to two minutes).
3. Use continuers to reinforce you are listening.
4. Paraphrase the history to show you are concerned to get the clinical history right and that you have listened to their story.
5. Use the question "What is it that worries you most?" to redirect a tangential history.
6. Use empathy when appropriate (e.g., "I'm sure that must be really tough for you").

THE PHYSICIAN EXAM

Typically, physicians don't speak to patients during a physical exam. We have learned that patients today want to know what you are doing and what you are finding. It is no longer acceptable for a nurse to measure a patient's blood pressure and turn her back on the patient to write it down, without commenting on what the numbers are. The more information we can provide to the patient regarding our findings correlates with patient-perceived value in the appointment. The physical exam is the perfect opportunity to exceed expectations without having to work any harder. Simply, think out loud.

The amount of information we can provide to the patient regarding our findings correlates with the patient-perceived value in the appointment.

As you conduct an examination, you will find the opportunity for a variety of comments, including:

- "I am going to listen to your heart and lungs now. You are moving air well and your lung fields sounds are clear. Your heart sounds are normal; I don't hear any murmurs or heart valve problems."
- "I feel no lymph node swelling or enlargement, your thyroid is normal size, and I hear no bruits over your internal carotid artery. A bruit is a sound a blood vessel can make if it is narrowed with plaque."
- "Your spleen and liver are normal size and everything in the abdominal area appears to be normal."

Simply conveying this information to patients during the course of the exam accomplishes a number of important objectives. First, it gives the patient a sense of the relatively large information gathered by the touch of expert hands. Second, it conveys completeness and comprehensiveness of your evaluation. Third, it positions the physician well in terms of our ability to extract information through our training and experience. Of course, we all know that a "normal" physical exam does not assure or even predict health and well-being, and this also must be clearly communicated to patients. Physical exam findings must be taken in context of all other subjective and objective patient information.

When physicians do provide explanations of the physical exam findings for patients, it will often create a response along the lines of, "How in the world can you tell all that in just a few seconds?" When this is skillfully done and presented to patients, succinctly and clearly, it is very impressive to them. The beauty of this tactic is that it is simply a conveyance of what we are already doing.

Like obtaining the history, when you conduct the physical exam for patients, it conveys completeness and a good faith effort to find a source or cause for symptoms. You are positioned in a way to create higher clinical effectiveness. Greater clinical effectiveness is fundamentally generated through establishing credibility through clinical thoroughness and the communication of information to patients in terms they can understand.

Key Learning Points—The Physician Exam

1. Providing information on physician exam findings conveys thoroughness and a diligent effort to find the cause of a problem.
2. Review your physical exam findings as you perform the exam.
3. The more information you provide to patients about themselves, the greater value for the visit in the eyes of patients.

PROVIDING PATIENT INFORMATION

Perhaps the most important clinical element to our patient visit is the explanation of medical information to patients. In fact, the most important determinant in the value of the visit rides on the patient's ability to understand our explanations of the diagnosis, treatment, medications, and lifestyle recommendations. Sharing medical data with the patient,[38] discussion of treatment effects,[39] increased time on health education,[40] and summarization of findings[41] have all correlated with improved patient outcomes. Unfortunately, it also is known that patients remember less than half of what physicians tell them just after a visit.[42] When developing techniques that facilitate conveyance of information, it is important to remember several important points:

• Patients will judge us as clinicians by our ability to *explain* a medical diagnosis, treatment, medication, or lifestyle change.

- The best treatment plan or most brilliant diagnosis DOES NOT MATTER if the patient does not understand it.
- Clear physician communication techniques improve patient recall of directions, improve patient satisfaction, and improve adherence to medical regimens.

Given these truths, how is this best done? A guide to doing this requires several proactive commitments from physicians as we develop tools to drive the effectiveness of what we do. The following are simple steps to getting this done for every patient, every time.

1. Every diagnosis, treatment, medication, or lifestyle change that you provide to any patient requires a simple explanation.

2. Drop the lingo. The communication gap often begins as the physician utilizes vocabulary that the patient doesn't understand.

3. Once you have provided patients information, query the patients for their understanding.

4. After each explanation to patients, ask, "Now, is there any more information you would need on that?" Patients then have an opportunity to ask any additional questions, but more importantly, they have the opportunity to say, "I've got it."

5. Be specific. When you provide specific directions, compliance and understanding improve. Telling patients to exercise 30 minutes five times a week is better than saying, "Get some exercise."

6. We often will see the same diagnosis, use the same medications, and offer similar treatment plans over and over again. Work on simple, clear, complete explanations for common problems. Most conditions and medications can be done in just a few sentences, if done well.

7. Ask patients to repeat the treatment plan as they understand it, which solidifies understanding and identifies any need for further explanation.

The days of providing a prescription, followed by, "Take this twice a day for the next 10 days," then walking out of the exam room are well behind us, and will assure dissatisfaction, loss of loyalty, noncompliance, and compromised clinical outcomes. **Providing clinical information should be considered a must-have behavior for physician performance.**

Key Learning Points—Providing Patient Information

1. Explanation of diagnosis and treatment plans is amongst the most important element of the patient visit.
2. Effective communication improves recall of directions, compliance, and patient satisfaction.
3. Every condition and plan must include a simple explanation.
4. All explanations must be followed by query of the patients for their understanding.
5. Ask patients to repeat the plan as they understand it to ensure their understanding and identify areas needing further explanation.

PATIENT/PHYSICIAN COLLABORATION

Listening, performing a careful physical exam, and clearly explaining clinical findings and treatment plans are in excess of what most physicians do for patients currently. The most exceptional and clinically successful physicians are those who have developed specific techniques to collaborate with patients. Proactive collaboration is a means for physicians to assure unsurpassed patient loyalty and word of mouth that will create patients who will do anything, including making financial sacrifices, to stay with them.

More importantly, collaborative decision making between patient and physician promotes self-management and improves management of chronic disease. Providing information alone is not sufficient to influence human behavior. A meta-analysis of 12 randomized controlled trials on information-only programs for asthmatic adults found no improvement in the number of physician visits, hospitalization rates, frequency of asthma attacks, or medication usage.[43] Simply telling patients what to do does not foster patient responsibility or behavioral change and is clinically less effective.

Effective collaboration with patients drives the ability and probability for patients to care for themselves. How people self-manage their chronic diseases can be at least as important as the actual health care they receive. Collaboration is not about physicians simply telling patients what to do to improve their health, but rather creating a shared responsibility for making and carrying out health-related decisions.

Collaboration is not about physicians simply telling patients what to do to improve their health, but rather creating a shared responsibility for making and carrying out health-related decisions.

Collaboration and shared decision making have been widely demonstrated to improve measures of chronic disease management. In a study comparing the ability to improve diabetes management as measured by HemoglobinA1c, two groups were compared. The first group received didactic information only in regards to diabetes management. The other group was provided a simple 20-minute intervention designed to increase their participation in decision making as well as information gathering from their physician. The intervention group showed a statistically significant drop in HemoglobinA1c levels compared to those receiving didactic information alone, even though there were no differences in diabetes knowledge between the two groups.[44]

In another recent study, researchers concluded, "Enhancing patient/physician communication and sharing decision making have been shown to result in greater patient satisfaction, adherence to treatment plans, and improved health outcomes. The consistency of these studies' findings of improved physiologic outcomes and reported health status is impressive."[45]

Collaboration is a process between the physician and patient to consider the available information about the medical problem, including available treatment options, and proceed with treatment plans based upon the patient's preference for health status and outcomes. Unfortunately, current medical practices rarely engage collaborative decision making. In a study of 1,000 physician visits, the patient did not participate in decisions 91 percent of the time.[46]

So, in the midst of the hectic 15-minute visit, how does a physician create collaboration with patients? A number of simple approaches have been found effective in creating a collaborative, cooperative partnership that drives patient satisfaction, compliance, and clinical outcomes.

1. **Goal Setting**—Create specific goals for clinical measures. This must be done with active patient participation and agreement. Ask patients what they think they can achieve. Achievement of patient-selected goals has been shown to be more effective than physician-selected goals.[47]

2. **Establish Collaboration**—The physician must take a moment when creating treatment recommendations to firmly establish a cooperative, collaborative effort toward a clinical goal. This is done by a dialogue that establishes that patients understand and are comfortable with the treatment plan, and if they have any reservations or wor-

ries that could result in noncompliance. Here is what can be said to the patient to help establish collaboration:

    a.   Does this treatment plan sound reasonable to you?

    b.   Do you have any worries or reservations about our plan?

    c.   I want to make sure we are on the same page in regards to our treatment plan.

    d.   This treatment plan works only if you are comfortable with it and are willing to do it. Do you have any reservations or concerns that would prevent you from taking this medication?

These are simple interactive strategies that make patients feel they are active participants and owners of their treatment plan. Collaborative strategies foster patient responsibility, promote self-management, and drive superior clinical outcomes and should be a component of all physician/patient interactions.

Key Learning Points—Collaboration with Patients

1. Establishing collaboration with patients improves compliance, outcomes, and patient satisfaction.
2. Collaboration can be established by asking patients if they have any reservations or concerns in regard to a treatment plan.
3. Collaboration is about specifically soliciting patient input regarding the treatment plan going forward.

PATIENT FOLLOW-UP

When a medical visit is completed, it is important that patients have a clear picture as to what will happen next. Tell patients what will be happening in very specific terms. The fundamental issu[e] must be clarified for patients before they leave include:

1. When or if you need to see the patient back again

This follow-up can include a contingency, meaning if you treat a patient for a cough with symptomatic measures, let him know under what circumstances to return to see you. If a follow-up is necessary, let him know the exact time frame and the purpose of the next visit. "Let's arrange a follow-up in three months to be sure your blood sugars are staying under good control."

2. Informing of test results

When laboratory or diagnostic tests are ordered, patients must be told when and how they will be informed of test results. "No news is good news" is not only a dissatisfier in the eyes of patients, but it falls out of compliance of medical group regulatory requirements. Your practice must institute a means of informing patients of laboratory and diagnostic tests, and patients must have a clear understanding of when and how they will receive their results. An example would include:

"We will mail you a copy of your cholesterol results within the next two weeks. If there are any problems with your results, I will be giving you a call to review the findings."

3. When the physician needs to call to inform patients of results

It is recommended that physicians call patients directly for the following tests:

- Major radiographic test results, including ultrasounds, CT scans, and MRI images. These are tests that will often evaluate patients for potentially serious conditions, and patients want to hear from the ordering physician regarding results.
- Abnormal laboratories that require initiation of medical treatment. If a patient will require a statin, or the initiation of

thyroid replacement, the patient will have a host of questions that will need clarification. Your nurse will be placed in an awkward position of fielding issues and concerns from the patient that she may not be comfortable with. When specific treatment is necessary, the physician should make the call personally.

- Abnormal biopsy results: All patients with abnormal biopsy results should be called by the physician with a clear plan as to what will happen next.

4. Establishing follow-up with specialty physicians

If specialty consultation is necessary, the following must be clearly explained to the patient. The patient needs to know:

- The purpose of the consultation and what specific clinical issue you need assistance with.
- The expertise the consulting physician will bring to the case.
- You will remain active in the case and will be receiving information directly from the consulting physician reinforcing the perception of continuity of care involving a "team" of physicians.
- Your opinion as to the clinical talent and quality of the physician you have selected to render an opinion on the case. Positioning your colleagues well is critical to sustaining the care experience for the patient as they see different consulting physicians.

(See Chapter 4 for additional information on Specialty Physicians and Consultants)

5. When follow-up with a specialist requires a longer wait than the patient wants

A frequent frustration and dissatisfier for patients as they leave your office is the time required to obtain specialty consultations. We will see a patient, often several times, for a clinical issue that persists despite our clinical efforts, prompting specialty referral. You fill out the consult form and send it to your receptionist for scheduling, only to find out that it will be six weeks before the patient can be seen. This will frustrate most patients, and will often leave them feeling as though your concern for their clinical improvement is less than they feel it should be.

Here are tactics to pre-empt this patient perception, without actually having to solve the specialty access issue:

- Once a recommendation is made to see the specialist, decide on a time frame that you are comfortable with in terms of the consultation date.
- The majority of cases referred do not need to be seen immediately. For those cases, inform the patient that it will take some time to get in to see the specialist, and that you think that will be fine. Also, inform the patient that, should his condition change, he should call you, and you will be sure he is taken care of.
- Position your specialist well (manage up). Your sincere recommendation carries tremendous credibility from the patients who have entrusted you in their care. Let them know that the reason for the wait is the skill of the physician and he or she is "worth the wait."

The fundamental priority of the closing of the patient interaction is that it must be made clear what will be happening next. Everything from follow-up, return of laboratories or diagnostic tests, specialty consultation, or the timing of biopsy turnaround must be clearly communicated to the patient. More importantly, you must execute exactly what you say you will do. If you tell patients their labs will be mailed within two weeks, it must be done, every time. If you tell a patient a letter is going to go out regarding mammogram results, you must be sure that a system is in place such that it always happens.

Effectively managing patient expectations circumvents and prevents many of the frustrations patients often reference.

Key Learning Points—Patient Follow-up

1. All patients must leave a visit understanding exactly what it is that will happen next.

2. Provide clear follow-up on the timing and purpose of patients' upcoming visits.

3. Provide information regarding the timing of laboratory and radiographic tests and how the results will get to the patient.

4. Explain the purpose and timing for specialty consultation in terms of when, why, and who.

5. Position specialty physician colleagues well.

EFFECTIVE APPOINTMENT CLOSURE

Much like the initial moments of the physician/patient interaction drive a sustained first impression of the interaction, the last moments create the final impression for patients when they leave. The last few words you say to a patient can solidify an effective collaborative appointment, or they can undo much of the good work you did in the moments preceding. The objective of an effective appointment closure is to have patients leave with a clear understanding of their primary health concerns, a collaborative treatment plan in partnership with the physician, and clarity on what will happen next.

The objective of an effective appointment closure is to have patients leave with a clear understanding of their primary health concerns, a

collaborative treatment plan in partnership with the physician,
clarity on what will happen next, and an unwavering loyalty to a
physician who has provided exceptional care.

———————————————

Much of your work is done in terms of creating a clinically effective partnership, and these closing tools are a means to finishing strong.

Finishing the office visit:

- Briefly summarize what you have agreed upon in terms of the treatment plan.
- Briefly summarize the next steps.
- Query the patient… "Now, does this all sound reasonable to you?"
- Ask the patient… "Is there anything else I can do for you?"
- Finish with… "Great, I will see you in six months, and call me if anything changes or concerns arise in the interim."
- Close the appointment with a handshake or a hand on the shoulder. Never underestimate the importance of the human touch in health care.

Physicians telling patients to call them or inform them of notable clinical changes does several things. First, it rarely increases the likelihood that patients will actually call and follow up unnecessarily. Second, it creates the perception of continual partnership and availability of the treating physician for the patient. The "I am here for you should things go bad" platform from the physician creates patients who will never leave you and will tell their friends that you are simply the best.

Physicians can again become nervous when we speak of the prospect of actually saying, "Is there anything else I can do for you?"

at the end of the visit. What if the patient says yes? We find that when you deploy the techniques of history collection, communication of information with a query of patient understanding, an articulation of what will happen next, and a closing that summarizes the collaborative plan, almost none of your patients will hit you with the "Oh, by the way" that all of us dread.

Key Learning Points—Effective Appointment Closure

1. How you finish the appointment will leave the final impression for the patient visit.
2. Review the collaborative treatment plan.
3. Query the patient to assure they are in agreement and understand the go forward plan.
4. Ask the patient, "Is there anything else I can do for you?"
5. Finish with, "I will see you in six months, and call me if you have any questions or concerns in the interim."
6. Close the appointment with a handshake or a touch on the shoulder.

The tools to providing exceptional service to patients are the same tools that drive clinical understanding, compliance, and outcomes. Exceptional service is about providing better health care, being a better physician, and establishing a reputation for excellence in your community. The tools provided work, and creating the patient experience remains a matter of their consistent implementation. Every patient, every time.

CHAPTER 4:
SPECIALTY AND CONSULTANT PHYSICIANS

The fundamental tools to creating the patient experience that drives patient loyalty, creates physician reputation, facilitates clinical effectiveness, and exceeds patient expectations are similar, regardless of specialty. These are techniques that foster trust and allow greater physician influence over what patients do for you and for themselves. Some noteworthy differences in approach do exist between primary and specialty care. These areas include specialty care access, referral efficiency, first impressions in specialty care, collaborative techniques, and creating continuity.

SPECIALTY CARE ACCESS

Poor access to specialty physicians significantly impacts patient satisfaction. Systems in which patients have to wait for weeks or months to see specialty physicians will diminish patient satisfaction with the entire medical group. If a referral is regulated by primary care, and a referral is denied, patients are significantly less satisfied with the group. Patients who experience ongoing access difficulties are more likely to leave the plan and less likely to recommend the group to a friend.[48]

Prior to patients ever getting to specialty care, they are often left frustrated and irritated at having to wait so long for appointments. The testimony of specialty physicians is often, "How in the world am

I supposed to make this patient happy when I can't do his total knee replacement for six months?" Access problems seem pervasive in many multispecialty group environments, and if you wait for this problem to be "solved" prior to making commitments to improve the patient experience, you may be waiting forever. Solving access issues is a major operational undertaking, and solutions do not necessarily include just hiring more physicians. The question is: *What can medical groups do now to improve the patient experience without having to wait for a solution that may take years to realize?*

Here are tactics to minimize the adverse impact that poor access can have amongst specialty physicians:

- When primary care physicians make referrals, it is important to manage the patient's expectations.
  - "I am going to have you see our cardiologist, Dr. Smith, to assist us in management of your atrial fibrillation. Dr. Smith is outstanding, and there is frequently a wait to get in to see him. I believe your condition is stable now, and I think the wait will be safe. Should your condition change, call me and we will be sure to take care of you. "
- Create an efficient referral process. Many conditions can be managed in primary care utilizing evidence-based clinical guidelines. Determine appropriate "referral criteria" for common problems. Specialty physicians often report that they would not have an access problem if the appropriateness of referrals improved.

SPECIALTY REFERRAL EFFICIENCY

An idealized referral process has a number of important components to improving the patient experience and clinical care. These include:

- When a referral is made, the patient and the specialty physician need to know the exact issue and question at hand. When patients don't know the pathway and purpose of their care, the sense of continuity diminishes. When the perception of continuity is disrupted, patients can begin to lose confidence in the team and clinical effectiveness is impacted.
- During a referral process, the referring physician must have a dedicated process to communicate the clinical question and the current work-up to the consulting physician.
- Prior to walking into the room with the patient, the specialty physician needs to have access and knowledge of all previous care.

SPECIALTY CARE FIRST IMPRESSIONS

Specialty physicians are in a position in which longitudinal relationships with patients may not exist. Physicians consulting on a patient may see the patient once or twice, leaving minimal opportunity to recover from lost service opportunities. A bad first impression may be enough to compromise a specialist's ability to effectively influence and manage the course of treatment.

Creating a first impression for patients seeing specialty physicians has several unique elements. The prescriptive first impression described in Chapter 3 applies here as well. Introduction, handshake, smile, sitting, and good eye contact are all essential for every physician for every patient encounter.

Additional behaviors for specialty encounters include:

- Specialty physicians need to state in early introductions the reason for the visit, as communicated by the primary care physician.
- Confirm with patients that they concur with the purpose of the visit.

- Briefly review the course of care as you have reviewed it, including your summary of the diagnostic work-up and therapeutic trials to date.
- Spend time telling patients your expertise and experience. In dealing with referral-related conditions, patients begin to place more weight and importance on clinical expertise, and you need to articulate this.
- Position primary care physicians well. Assume that patients have a strong relationship with their primary care physicians, and speaking well of them will create allegiance to you.

COLLABORATIVE TECHNIQUES FOR SPECIALISTS

Creating treatment collaboration is different for specialties than for primary care physicians. The reason for this difference is that several physicians are involved in the care of the patient, and implementation of treatment requires assurance that all involved physicians are in concurrence. If the consulting physician makes a recommendation in stark contrast to a trusted primary care physician, confidence in both can be compromised.

Here are tactics for specialty physicians to create collaboration with patients and other treating physicians:

- Communicate to patients that their primary care physician is asking for help to best manage their case, but you will continue to work together.
- Communicate to patients that you will be providing all information, thoughts, and recommendations to their physician.
- If there is a marked change in the management of a clinical problem, explain the reason for the change.
- Never criticize another physician's treatment approach in the presence of the patient. Everyone loses when this is done.

- With any new treatment recommendation, query patients for their understanding and their acceptance of this approach.
- Always utilize and leverage the relationship patients have with their primary care physician to improve your ability to establish trust.

On many occasions I have seen patients return to me from specialty consultations in which collaborative steps were not taken by the consulting physicians. These were cases in which the reason for the consultation conveyed by me to the patient was not acknowledged or referenced by the consultant, and where the consulting physician made no reference to any of the history or work-up the patient had gone through to date. In addition, there was no proactive effort to connect care to the primary physician who had managed the patient for years. These patients would return to me feeling disconnected from a previously articulated path of care, with little positive to say about the consulting physician.

CREATING CONTINUITY

The challenge of handing patients from physician to physician for complex medical cases is important, not only in terms of the patient experience, but also to ensure the safety and clinical outcomes of patients. The above techniques to establish and communicate collaboration with patients are essential to the perception of coordinated care. Distinguished specialists in the community who have the reputation for clinical excellence and who have physician referral bases that predictably and preferentially refer to them, are the physicians who establish continuity with the patient and referring physician.

Here are tactics for specialty physicians to exceed expectations of patients and referring physicians:

- When a specialty physician completes a consultation, deliver the clinical note by secured e-mail. Referring physicians can see your recommendations the day of the consult, and e-mail can serve as a two-way communication device. A dictation sent in the mail is dated, takes time, and doesn't utilize widely available technologies.
- Let patients know that you will be providing your recommendations to their primary physician on the day of your consult, creating a sense that there is a team of physicians in close communication, collaborating in their treatment.
- If the consultant is assuming the care of the patient, convey to the patient that you will be keeping the primary care physician informed on the course of care.

The ideal consultant interaction is one that provides clear clinical expertise, communication and collaboration with the patient, and prompt feedback and exchange with the primary care physician, and leaves the patient and the referring physician with the sense that they have added a valuable player to the team. To make this happen, specialty physicians need to understand and implement service efforts, and the extent to which they will predict compliance to recommended treatments. Equally important, specialty physicians' continued referrals from physicians will be predicted by what patients say about them as they follow up with their own physicians. When patients return from a consult saying, "That doctor didn't know why I was there, didn't explain things, and didn't know anything about the things we had already tried…why did you send me to him?" will equally frustrate the patient and referring physician. It takes just one patient comment like this to change what referring physicians do going forward.

Effective consultation is equally dependent on the primary care physician. Primary care physicians need to provide intelligent, appropriate work-ups within the scope of their practice. Referring physicians need to ask and communicate specific clinical questions of a consultant, and manage the patient's expectations for access-related issues. Primary care physicians need to position consultant colleagues positively in the eyes of patients, and to remain owners of the care, maintaining responsibility and advocacy for the patient as they move from primary to specialty care.

Key Learning Points—Specialty and Consultant Physicians

1. Fundamental service tools apply to specialty physicians as well as primary care physicians, including knocking, introduction, handshake, eye contact, and sitting.

2. Referring physicians must minimize the negative impact of poor specialty access by managing patients' expectations.

3. Position consultant physicians well in terms of clinical expertise and experience to convey that they are "worth the wait."

4. Create clinical "referral criteria" for common problems to minimize unnecessary referrals.

5. All referrals need to come with a standardized communication, including the clinical question at hand, work-up to date, and previous therapeutic trials.

6. The patient needs to be told by the referring physician the exact purpose of the visit.

7. The consultant needs to communicate to the patient the purpose of the visit, and review the work-up to date to establish continuity as it was communicated by the referring physician.

8. Consultant physicians need to review with the patient the expertise they bring to the case.

9. Create collaboration with the patient in regards to changes in diagnostic or therapeutic approaches.

10. Consultant physicians need to tell patients they will be in communication with the primary care physician regarding the course of treatment, preferably communicating information the same day utilizing secured e-mail.

CHAPTER 5:

SERVICE RECOVERY FOR PHYSICIANS

Service recovery is a process to recover when things go wrong. No matter how good you and your organization become, circumstances and situations arise that result in unmet patient expectations. The response of your organization to these unmet expectations is one of the most important tools to hardwire into every layer of your organization. A single unrecovered service is not only a source of negative word of mouth in your community, but the wrong thing happening to the wrong patient can be a viable threat to the reputation of your entire organization. In the age and the availability of rapid dissemination of information on the Internet, even the best of organizations are at risk from angry customers and angry patients.

In the age and availability of rapid information dissemination, the wrong thing happening to the wrong patient can be a viable threat to the reputation of your entire organization.

British Airways has implemented an aggressive service recovery program. Their program has resulted in a doubling of customer retention of those who complain, as well as a 200 percent increase in return on investment for money spent on service recovery. Industry leaders have replicated these findings many times over. When service recovery is done right, it works. In fact, a well-recovered service leaves the customer more satisfied than if nothing had gone wrong in the first place. Customers who are very satisfied with service provided will tell three to four people about their experience. Customers who are very dissatisfied with care and services will tell *five times that number of people*.

When the care of the patient is involved, by far the most effective player in the service recovery team is the physician. A physician who proactively intervenes for the good of the patient when things have gone poorly is very powerful. The elements of service recovery that work for physicians are simple, logical, and prescriptive. There is little negotiation in terms of how this should be done. When service recovery is done on "our terms" with disregard for the patient perspective, it will not work and can often inflame an already difficult situation. Patient complaints in the medical group setting are associated with malpractice risk.[49] Service recovery is critical to minimize liability exposure.

Prior to articulating the tools for service recovery, it is important to know when this action is necessary. The most important requisite for effective service recovery is to recognize when things have gone badly, prior to your patient storming up to the receptionist counter complaining that he has been waiting 45 minutes. The most common reason for service recovery failure is the failure to recognize that we fell short in the first place. The following are proactive opportunities for service recovery before having to respond to a specific complaint. Remember, only 10 percent of those who are dissatisfied with service will complain about it to you.

The most common reason for service recovery failure is the failure to recognize that we fell short in the first place. Only 10 percent of those who are dissatisfied with service will complain.

Opportunities where service recovery should be initiated:

- Patients waiting more than 20 minutes for an appointment
- Patient calls not being returned on the day they were placed
- Patients coming to pick up a prescription or form at your office and it wasn't done
- Diagnostic study results not returned to patient in the expected time frame
- Patients' appointments having to be cancelled and rescheduled due to physician availability

It is advised to develop organizational standards as to when service recovery is engaged, and to have this standard embedded in the training and expectations of staff and physicians. Your staff, to as great an extent as possible, needs to be empowered to solve the problem on the spot, without having to "get someone" who actually knows what they are doing. When problems are "deflected," it tends to reinforce the patient perception that we may really be as incompetent as we appear. At The Ritz-Carlton, every staff member, from the groundskeeper to bell captain, has an open $2,000 tab to solve customer-related problems immediately, without authorization from anyone.[50] Service recovery as a cultural trait is a trademark of great organizations.

Here are sequential steps in effective service recovery:

1. **Apologize.** A blameless apology where you are simply and honestly sorry that this happened to this patient. Saying you are sorry conveys empathy and concern without agreeing or disagreeing with the facts of the situation. Research has repetitively demonstrated that an apology is the first thing that dissatisfied customers want to hear.

2. **Let the patient speak.** Bring the patient to a private area, sit, and let the patient speak without interruption.

3. **Validate.** Stating that you realize how frustrating this must be is very effective in reducing patient anger.

4. **Correct the issue.** When a patient brings forward a complaint, the organization must act swiftly to resolve the issue. The physician usually is in a position where this can be done easily if the cited issue is related to the care of the patient.

5. **Take action.** Complaints that arise from patients are opportunities to improve. A great organization is one that responds promptly to mistakes and creates an accountability trail by which to ensure that the same errors don't continue to arise. Some organizations have used a log to register the complaint and to document resolution as an effort to create steps to reduce mistake recurrences. If the same mistakes continue to arise in the same departments, leaders must be held accountable to correct this.

6. **Follow up with the patient.** This is the step that will differentiate your organization from everyone else that implements service recovery measures. If you solve the problem, but don't profile the solution to the patient, you may not win the patient back. A next-day follow-up phone call to ensure and communicate sufficient resolution will usually suffice, and should be included in the service recovery closure.

Physicians and nurses may respond to a directive of service recovery with a concern that some patients are so ridiculous in their demands that nothing we ever do will make them happy. This does happen, and despite well-executed policies, patients can leave unhappy. In reality, most patients are nice, reasonable people, and believe we have done something that fell short. Their perception is our reality.

Well-executed service recovery retains patients, improves patient satisfaction, reduces malpractice exposure, and drives market share. It is a necessity for excellence and it is something that should be done at every level of the organization.

Perhaps the most important impact of promptly and quickly resolving conflict with patients is the ability to realign the patient and the physician toward a shared therapeutic goal. Effective health care can never be provided when the patient and physician are in opposition. Opposition creates distrust and anger, and establishes a physician/patient experience that makes patients leave and physicians burn out. There is nothing more emotionally exhausting than dealing with patients who are frustrated and angry with you and your staff as a result of an operational or service shortfall. Skills and tools for service recovery will transform the patient experience for the better. Equally important, effective recovery can lift a troublesome burden for physicians as we continue to strive to do the right thing.

Key Learning Points—Service Recovery for Physicians

1. Physicians are the most effective personnel to deal with unmet patient expectations.

2. The failure to recognize service shortfalls is the most common reason for service recovery failure.

3. Create organizational "indications" for service recovery initiation.

4. Empower and train staff to "solve" the problem, without having to "get someone else who knows what they are doing."

5. Steps in Service Recovery:

   Step 1. Apologize (blameless): "I'm sorry this happened."

   Step 2. Let the patient speak without interruption.

   Step 3. Validate the patient: "I know how frustrating this must be for you."

   Step 4. Correct the issue at hand; fix the problem immediately.

   Step 5. Take action to prevent recurrent similar problems from arising.

   Step 6. Profile the solution to the patient.

6. Effective service recovery improves patient satisfaction, reduces malpractice risk, and drives market share.

CHAPTER 6:

SOLUTIONS TO DIFFICULT PATIENT SITUATIONS

Difficult clinical situations are frustrating and taxing to even the most experienced physicians. These situations are time consuming and place the entire health care team on edge. Prescriptive tactics for navigation of these situations are important in sustaining service and clinical excellence. The fact is, many physicians have not learned tactics for dealing with these clinical situations and the physician response is often maladaptive and nonproductive, escalating the physician/patient conversation from a minor disconnect, to an aggravating exchange for the physician and the patient.

This chapter will explore a number of clinical situations that physicians will see every day, and will provide prescriptive responses to help the physician, as well as the patient.

SITUATION 1:

A patient comes to the office and demands a medically unnecessary test.

This is the most frequently cited frustration by physicians in terms of sources for physician/patient conflict. The scenario may include something as simple as a healthy female requesting a CA-125 ovarian cancer-screening test, to a patient with lumbar pain requesting an MRI scan, even prior to conservative management. In any case, the physician and the patient are set in opposition, and the tussle begins.

You must navigate this so that in the end you:

- Do the right thing medically
- Create a collaborative consensus with the patient
- Leave the patient satisfied
- Leave the physician satisfied

Here is how this can be done. Let's take the MRI case as an example. A 35-year-old male comes in with four days of severe, non-radicular lumbar pain after digging some ditches for his sprinkler system. Only on day four is he able to move enough to get to your office. He has been on ibuprofen with little relief. He has no history of protracted lower back pain, and no systemic symptoms. His physical exam reveals only peri-lumbar tenderness. He insists on an MRI scan, and won't leave until you order one.

RESPONSE TO A DEMANDED, UNNECESSARY TEST

1. Conduct a complete history and physical exam, assuring that nothing will be missed and conveying to the patient that you have thoroughly evaluated the medical complaint.
2. Clearly explain the diagnosis with clear anticipated outcomes and timelines for the patient.
3. Validate the diagnosis with phrases like:
   "A sprained lumbar spine with spasm can be extremely painful, and I can understand your concern and desire to get to the bottom of this immediately."
4. Pre-empt the test demand by clearly and simply explaining what it is the test can and can't do, and what the medical literature states as to the reasons or criteria for obtaining the test.

5. Tell the patient that you may end up ordering the test, but under what exact circumstances and timeline you would be prompted to do so.

6. Provide a clear therapeutic plan and what you expect to occur from this intervention.

7. Finish strong with a statement that aligns you and the patient to the same goal, and provides patient confidence he is in expert hands. For example:

"I know you are very concerned about your back, and I am here to give you the best and most current medical treatment possible. You have a back muscle strain with spasm that is causing your pain. I am going to prescribe a pain medication and a muscle relaxer to break this cycle for you. I will arrange to have you see the physical therapist in the next three days to assist you as well. I have treated this type of condition hundreds of times and we will get you through this. I know you wanted me to order an MRI scan. I can assure you that the MRI scan will not provide any information that we don't already know by your examination. Additionally, extensive research has been done on back pain and when MRI scans are helpful. I will be happy to order one for you when I think it will help us make better decisions. I give you an 80 percent chance of being significantly better within two weeks and I want you to call if you are not improving. One thing that is really important, though, is that you are comfortable with the plan and that you and I are on the same page. Does this plan sound reasonable to you?"

Done well, the above steps almost always will get you and the patient realigned and wanting the same thing. In navigating this successfully, always remember:

• Everything is done in the spirit of doing the best thing for the patient, as opposed to defending a position of not ordering a requested test. If a patient senses an oppositional position from you, your words will fall on deaf ears.

- Never "just order the test." This is the "adaptive" strategy that many physicians engage and they are mystified that their patients are still not satisfied. If there is any sense that you participated in the "…fine, I'll just order your test that you don't need so you'll stop bugging me" game, they will lose respect for you as a clinician. The patient will leave without getting what he or she really desired, which is an answer and communication regarding a very troubling clinical situation.

- Never order a test that can be harmful to a patient, when it is clearly not indicated. We will use this argument for young, healthy patients who come in requesting treadmills in the absence of risk factors or symptoms. Inform them why and how this test can do them more harm than good, and you will not subject them to that risk. In our experience, this approach works nearly every time.

- Remember, peace of mind may be a reasonable indicator to order an "unnecessary" test. Sometimes patients, despite going through all the outlined steps, continue to worry excessively about something that is being missed. If their fear is disproportionate to findings, ask them what their greatest worry is in regards to their symptoms. You may find a simple issue to which you can provide clarity. If you can't discover an underlying fear, order the test. Let them know that their ability to sleep at night and them being at "peace" is as important as anything, and that you are content with those reasons.

- Always do and say things that are for the good of patients, creating partnership, trust, and collaboration. If you do, they will almost always do what you think is best.

SITUATION 2:

A patient comes in with ten problems and demands they all be taken care of today.

If a physician is beginning to run behind, one of these situations is enough to ruin an entire day. The patient who somehow thinks we can manage, let alone document, examine, and provide information and treatment on a prohibitively long problem list is a patient who creates anxiety and dread for physicians. The percentage of patients who do this is relatively small, but again, it doesn't take many to drain vigor and enthusiasm from even the most seasoned physicians.

Here are strategies to combat this situation:

- Tell patients how long the appointment is. Most patients don't realize how long they have with you.
- Use a patient agenda (see Best Practices, Chapter 11) to create a manageable priority list for your visit.
- If you see a list that the patient brings in, swing your chair around and go over it together.
- Let patients know that you are most concerned about doing the right thing for them, and in order to do the best job, you can cover only the three or four most important issues today because it takes some time to do it right.
- If a patient is a chronic consumer of your time, book 30 minutes whenever that patient calls in (though don't let the patient know).
- Again, always say and do things that are conveyed in a way that your primary concern is doing what's best for them. When you make that case convincingly, patients will respond by being more respectful of your time and willing to comply with practice time limits.

SITUATION 3:

A patient comes to you seeking narcotic refills beyond what you think is medically necessary.

This is a source of significant conflict between physicians and patients. How is this navigated to where the right thing is done, and the patient leaves on the same page with the treating physician?

First, this will not be a lesson in drug seeking recognition, but how to communicate with patients who have a tendency to always seem to be in clinical situations where they are asking for controlled drugs.

Here are strategies to assist in doing the right thing for patients who may want something from you that you are rightfully reluctant to provide.

- Again, perform a complete history and physical exam to get as good a sense of pain medication requirements as a physician can. Specifically quantify and document patient's pain using a pain scale.
- Many physicians don't prescribe narcotic medications during a patient's first visit. State this clearly to patients if this is your policy.
- If the patient seems to be asking for excessive refills of narcotic medications, let the patient know that you are concerned about his ongoing requirements for narcotics and you need to see him to determine why this has gone on longer than expected.
- If concerns for drug seeking behavior persist after your re-evaluation, then you need to have the following conversation with the patient:
  - "I am here to do the right thing for you, and I am concerned that we may be creating an additional, more serious problem by continuing to prescribe controlled

drugs. Continuing to write these medications would be a tremendous disservice to you as my patient and we need to look at other ways of managing your pain."

- ° Drug seekers may simply leave your practice at this point. You have not accused them of anything, but created a case that they may become a "victim" of the medication, which is a much tougher point for a drug seeker to argue.
- If longer-term narcotic medications become necessary by your best clinical assessment, then consider the following:
  - ° A narcotic contract signed by the patient that includes the risks of the medication and that the patient will receive narcotics from a single pharmacy and physician. Make it clear within your contract that violation of the signed contract is grounds for patient termination.

SITUATION 4:

A patient arrives late and demands to be seen.

Very few patients arrive to the clinic late "on purpose." The majority have an unforeseen event and feel terrible and frustrated about arriving past their appointment time. Patients should be treated on the assumption that this circumstance holds true, and shouldn't be punished by poor service and disrespect by you or your staff. My philosophy is to see all patients, regardless of when they arrive. We're here; they're here. It makes no sense to send them away and rebook into an already tight schedule to do what you can do now. It works better for you and the patient to assume this policy.

Additionally, you never know whom you are going to be sending home. Recently, the son of a prominent leader in our organization arrived 20 minutes late for a visit, after being told the wrong site for his appointment. The policy within our organization is when a patient is over 20 minutes late, it is the physician's discretion to see the patient or not. In this case, the patient was not seen, and it was made clear to many of us what it is like from the patient's standpoint to be "sent home" after arriving late. No one wins.

The following are suggestions to maintain workflow when patients arrive late:

- See patients who have arrived on time first.
- Inform late patients that you will be working them into the schedule, and they may need to wait a bit, informing them specifically of wait times.
- If excessively late, inform the patient that the physician may need to do an abbreviated visit today, and can rebook if there are complicated issues that will be time consuming.
- If the patient is a repeat offender and is habitually late, then you need to create accountability. If he comes late again, have him rebook due to arriving late. He will arrive on time the next visit.

Again, construct the patient experience so that it is patient centered and designed to meet their needs. When patients' needs are met, they become more understanding, more gracious, more thankful, and better patients who are happier with their care.

How you and your organization deal with traditionally difficult situations can be a benchmark of performance under strain. Nobody likes dealing with these situations and it is easier to provide exceptional care and service when difficulties are not present, but it is more important to have hardwired behaviors when the stakes rise or when the prospect for confrontation mounts.

The directive for any potential conflict with a patient is that it must not be a conflict. This is not to be confused with giving patients whatever they want. Techniques have to be engaged knowingly and proactively to achieve alignment between physicians and patients. Exceptional health care can be delivered in no other way.

CHAPTER 7:

SERVICE IMPLEMENTATION TO PHYSICIANS—A STEPWISE APPROACH

The physician's ability to provide exceptional care and ensure clinical outcomes, partnership, and collaboration with patients will be a function of what the physician does for the patient in the exam room. The tools provided in Chapter 3 are effective, and physician performance simply remains a matter of implementation and consistency. Equally important, the sustainability and growth of the physician effort and commitment is dependent on the medical group culture in which the physicians work. In order to create broad, sustained physician behavioral change, physicians must see tangible evidence that service efforts will make the care provided by them better and more efficient. Physicians must see that a commitment to service will improve patient satisfaction, drive market share, retain staff, and create a reputation of excellence. Equally important, physicians must see and hear that service excellence within the organization is a critical path item and a principal strategic priority. If the service effort is not conveyed as important, the physicians won't see it as important and will be slower to engage the organizational mission.

In the end, how this service implementation effort is executed will determine your organization's ability to change, and whether physicians become your most loyal allies or your greatest barrier to organizational excellence.

STEP 1: PHYSICIAN LEADERSHIP COMMITS TO EXCELLENCE

An organizational decision and commitment to creating the best place to work, the best place to practice medicine, and the best place to receive care is a massive one. When making this decision, there can be no wavering, no hesitation, no reservation, and all levels of leadership must know full well that this is going to take extraordinary effort and time.

In the medical group environment, physician leadership must be willing to lead constituent physicians hand in hand with your administrative leadership as a unified effort. Physicians are the perceived leaders of your organization for those doing the work of patient care, and their visibility and support in this effort is a necessity.

Individual physician behavioral change does not occur in a vacuum. Behavioral change begins to occur when a medical group communicates a vision for group and individual success through the consistent execution of service and clinical excellence. Individual physician engagement and change are more probable when the strategic priorities and mission are communicated to physicians by respected physician leaders, and they understand that their role is central to success.

So what does it mean to lead a commitment to excellence for physician leaders? When making a decision for a commitment to service and operational excellence, the following points must be acknowledged:

- Physician leadership must be made up of high performers in the organization, who are respected by colleagues for their integrity and conduct within the group, who possess the ability to influence others.

- Physician leaders must understand the dynamics of the current consumer-driven medical marketplace, the forces that drive patient health care decisions, and what specifically their group will need to deliver to grow market share.

- Physician leaders must lead, and not follow this effort. This commitment is foundational to how care is delivered to patients; therefore, physician leadership needs to make this an organization priority, not a peripheral project "administration is working on."

- Physician leaders must, in time, present this effort to constituent physicians as an expectation, not a request.

- Physician leadership should be involved with this commitment as early as possible. Do not wait to "get your house in order" prior to engaging physicians. Bringing physicians to the table at the inception of your organizational commitment will help create physician "ownership."

- Physician leadership must realize that they will encounter vocal resistance during this organizational betterment, and that they can't move forward without leaving a few behind.

- Physician leadership must stand with consensus on their platform of being the best. Leaders must be unified in their commitment to organizational excellence and make all decisions based on that platform. Individual physician agendas that run counter to the prevailing group mission must not change the direction or momentum of the effort.

- Physicians in leadership positions who criticize and undermine the organizational commitment to service can have a significant impact on the ability to create physicians' support, and must be realigned.

- Physician leaders must model the conduct and behaviors that they expect of their constituent physicians.

STEP 2: SELECT A PHYSICIAN CHAMPION
(The Physician "Fire Starter")

Once physician leaders make a commitment to lead your group to service and operational excellence, the need will arise for a physician Champion ("Fire Starter"). There are training, coaching, physician behavioral standards, and administrative collaborative efforts that will need to be coordinated, and a designated physician Fire Starter needs to lead this effort.

Who communicates and coordinates the change effort and how it is done is critical for effective engagement of your physicians. Instilling and creating physician behavioral change is a challenging proposition, and to whom physicians listen is highly selective. It is very impactful when a respected colleague who does the same things, sees the same patients, and works as hard as anyone else, stands up and says:

"This is the right thing to do for our patients, the right thing to do for our staff, and the right thing for us to do. We will succeed by providing exceptional care to patients in the kind of collaborative, purposeful work environment that will make us the best..."

This message needs to be prominent, repetitive, and consistent, and it needs to come from every element of your organization, with your physician leadership and Fire Starter at the point. In order for your physician Fire Starter to have success in creating physician engagement and creating change, he or she must operate in the context of organizational support from department chairs, the board of directors, and respected physician leaders. Never send your physician Fire Starter out to initiate this effort with wavering or hesitant support. The physician will fail, and your chance to lead your group to become exceptional will be notably handicapped. It must be done right the first time.

So, whom do you select to be your physician "Fire Starter"? Here are "Fire Starter selection criteria" to provide guidance on who will best serve this role:

Physician Fire Starter Selection Criteria:

1. **High peer review:** To engage physician colleagues, your physician Fire Starter must be respected within the group. Internal peer review processes are a critical "first screen" for those who can lead this effort effectively.

2. **High patient satisfaction:** Your physician Fire Starter must model the behaviors that you seek to develop within your group.

3. **Strong collaborative abilities:** Your physician Fire Starter must be able to work cooperatively with physician and administrative leadership, nurses, and staff throughout the clinics. Excessively headstrong and noncompromising approaches are not effective.

4. **Strong communication skills:** Much of what a physician Fire Starter does involves speaking, teaching, training, and even inspiring. Your selected Fire Starter must be comfortable in this position. Though these responsibilities can be learned to a certain extent, if someone is terrified of public speaking, this is not a position for him or her.

5. **Commitment:** The most important thing to consider in making this selection is to find someone who is totally committed to the mission of making health care better for your medical group. It is a long journey that will never end, one that will be filled with progress as well as frustrations. Steadfastness and an unwillingness to ever give up is an absolute necessity.

After reviewing these "selection criteria," you may wonder if you have any physicians who fit this description. You probably have this physician in your midst; you just don't know it yet. When you select the right physician, and provide the training and support for effective leadership, you may be surprised at what your physician Fire Starter can become. With the right selection, and the appropriate training, you will likely have in your presence an impassioned leader driven to train, motivate, engage, and lead your physicians to organizational excellence.

STEP 3: DEFINE THE ROLE OF YOUR PHYSICIAN FIRE STARTER

A Fire Starter is an impassioned leader who is driven to make a difference. In the words of a great Fire Starter, Quint Studer, "Never underestimate the difference one person can make." The impact of a single physician on the operations and culture of a group can be significant when the right person is selected, the role is clarified, and organizational support is in place.

When selecting and launching a physician Fire Starter position within your group, it is important to have a guide as to what the scope and role of that position might be. Certainly, the role of the Fire Starter will be made by your organization in terms of your needs, but we will provide an outline of what some of these responsibilities and goals may look like.

Physician Fire Starter Responsibilities:

- Communicate the vision of service and operational excellence as foundational to medical organization success.
- Communicate with physician leadership the strategy and progress regarding physician performance improvement.
- Maintain service excellence as a principal strategic priority for physicians.
- Coordinate and conduct physician service excellence training.
- Develop patient satisfaction feedback that provides physicians their comparative performance and identifies opportunities for improvement.

- Coach low-performing physicians as measured by patient satisfaction.
- Collaborate with administrative leadership to assist with staff training.
- Create reward and recognition tools for high-performing physicians.
- Collaborate with physician leadership to create and implement behavioral standards for staff physicians.
- Monitor physician satisfaction to assure physicians' concerns are heard and addressed.

We suggest that the physician selected for this position have administrative time by which to initiate and lead these efforts. An agreement should be reached between the medical group and the physician regarding a fair monthly stipend commensurate with the time and value of these efforts. These are details that can be worked out within your own organization.

STEP 4: TRAIN YOUR PHYSICIAN FIRE STARTER

In order for your physician Fire Starter to be effective, not only do you have to select the right leader and provide vigorous organizational support, but, most importantly, you must train your Fire Starter to lead. Even high-performing physicians will not necessarily have the skill set to lead this effort effectively. High-performing physicians know how to take excellent care of patients and to get the best from their staff, but receive little training in physician leadership. When selected to lead this effort, one must assume the role of a student, learning all he or she can about drivers of patient satisfaction and physician satisfaction and predictors of physician behavioral change.

Here is a suggested curriculum for a new physician Fire Starter:

- "Bringing You and Your Organization to the Next Level" conducted by Quint Studer. This is an excellent overview of the core "Nine Principles®" of organizational change to drive results.
- "Good to Great" by Jim Collins. This detailed, research-based study explores how leaders and organizations obtain excellence and the specific determinants of greatness.
- "Nuts and Bolts of Emergency Medicine" led by Julie Kennedy, RN, and Jay Kaplan, MD, of Studer Group. This is a very helpful "practical application" of service and operational efforts in the emergency room and urgent care setting, and it applies easily to the medical group outpatient environment.
- Read every article and book available regarding physician leadership, the patient experience, and the physician's role in organizational performance.

This initial training will allow your physician Fire Starter to gain a vision and an outline to initiate strategic planning for engaging the physicians of your medical group. Once your physician Fire Starter has foundational training in the drivers of physician and organizational performance, the prospect of launching a campaign of service and operational excellence amongst the general physician staff will be much less daunting.

STEP 5: LAUNCH THE COMMITMENT TO EXCELLENCE AND TRAIN YOUR PHYSICIANS

After completing the steps outlined above, it is time to launch this commitment to excellence to your physicians. One thing should be made perfectly clear: You have one chance to do this. If it is not done well, you will lose credibility, and the effort to engage and lead your physicians to change will be compromised. We suggest that a launch be a dedicated event, with mandatory or "incentivized" attendance.

The following should be objectives of your launch:

- A clear statement that your group is committed to service excellence as a critical strategic priority in your organization.
- A concise review of how service excellence drives patient satisfaction, loyalty, market share, word of mouth referrals, reduced malpractice risk, improved compliance, improved clinical outcomes, improved physician satisfaction, and improved employee satisfaction. There simply is no other organizational effort that can yield this kind of return on physician investment.
- The physicians' role in this effort.
- Prescriptive tools on how physicians treat patients, staff and colleagues in an organization committed to service and operational excellence.

When designing this physician training program, you must integrate some key components that will allow this training to engage, inspire, and motivate your physicians to lay the foundation for engagement and sustainment of behavioral change.

Steps to Effective Physician Training:

1. **Profile the positive things about your medical group.** Even those groups that struggle with patient satisfaction will have successes within the organization. Generate pride in the institution. Remember, physicians are more inclined to "get on board" when vision and accomplishment are evident. State the mission of your organization and the unwavering commitment of your leadership to be the best.

2. **Create the "burning platform."** In order for physicians to become receptive to change, they need to understand why

change is necessary. Physicians must understand the data that is driving this effort. A compelling, clear presentation of your data will get your physicians to listen. Be prepared to defend your patient satisfaction tool, because that will arise, particularly if your scores are low. A predictor of an organization's ability to improve is the ability of an organization to be brutally honest with itself. Look candidly at your data, and pull no punches here to create the argument for change.

3. **Review the compelling evidence for service excellence.** The case for service is strong in the literature and has demonstrated that it will improve patient satisfaction and patient loyalty and reduce malpractice exposure. It will improve economic returns, patient care, clinical outcomes, and will ultimately drive physician satisfaction. Physicians need to hear this evidence in a way that makes them feel as though they must and want to proceed with the tools that will make it happen.

4. **Provide practical tools.** These prescriptive behaviors are best formatted into how physicians treat staff, patients, and each other within a new Culture of Excellence.

   a. **How Physicians Treat Staff**—Physicians will need guidance and training to understand how their treatment of staff will predict staff performance, loyalty, and retention, and will significantly affect the bottom line of the organization. More importantly, if physicians don't role model service, respect, and collaboration in the workplace, service excellence is unlikely to happen at the frontline.

   b. **How Physicians Treat Patients**—Physicians must implement simple prescriptive tools that work to drive service excellence and clinical effectiveness. (see Physician Service Tools, Chapter 3)

   c. **How Physicians Treat Each Other**—Physician satisfaction and professional fulfillment is tightly correlated to the relationships a physician has with colleagues.

Collaboration, cooperation, support, respect, friendship, and positioning each other well in the eyes of patients should be core values that are trained and expected of your staff physicians.

5. **Provide physician testimony.** An effective way to close training is to find a respected physician within your group to stand up and provide a personal testimony as to why this effort must be done. When physicians use the service and collaborative tools that work, and realize what happens to their practice when they dedicate themselves to making a difference for patients, the practice of medicine becomes fun again. The personal story of the difference these efforts make in the life of a colleague is compelling and can resonate with your physicians.

6. **Provide physicians the patient satisfaction data.** Following physician training, provide individualized patient satisfaction data to each of your physicians, including national comparative data. Providing this data to your physicians will serve as their starting point and will create a tangible profile of current physician performance.

The launch of this effort should be rehearsed and well thought out. Select a speaker who is experienced in the outpatient medical group arena and someone who is able to engage physicians, ideally a fellow physician. Your physician Fire Starter can host the event and work with the presenter to ensure that organizational objectives are met.

A successful physician training presentation on service and operational excellence is an excellent starting point to engaging your physicians, but it is not enough to sustain behavioral change. The tools provided to physicians need to be presented more than once, and they must be accompanied by ongoing support for these service efforts by the physician leadership. It must become apparent that implementation and effort for service excellence is evolving into a physician expectation, not a request.

STEP 6: MEASURE PHYSICIAN PERFORMANCE AND PROVIDE FEEDBACK

Once your commitment to service excellence has been clearly and repeatedly disseminated to your physicians, and tools and training are provided, the time comes to track and use patient satisfaction to drive performance. Patient satisfaction data is most effective when it is fully transparent within your organization, and this should be the ultimate goal of patient satisfaction measurement.

The process of providing physicians with patient satisfaction results must proceed in a stepwise fashion, depending on the maturation of the culture of your group. The data provided to physicians will be a function of which patient satisfaction vendor your organization utilizes.

The following represents one example of the progressive unveiling of data for physicians' performance toward patient satisfaction transparency.

1. Provide physicians individual, noncomparative data that simply gives raw numbers for each of the patient survey questions.
2. Provide physicians comparative data utilizing national percentile ranks that are generated from raw scores.
3. Provide internal medical group rank, both overall and where they stand within their own department.
4. "Unblind" their comparative results within their own departments, allowing physicians to see colleagues' performance within their own department.
5. "Unblind" all patient satisfaction results for all physicians within your medical group, so that all physician results are displayed for everyone to see.

Steps one through five may take one to two years to achieve, but it is clear that the best medical groups in the country are data transparent. The progressive unveiling of results requires an ongoing drumbeat from medical group physician leadership that the highest priority of your group remains service and clinical excellence. If your physicians continually hear this message, then the divulgence of scores will be consistent with the mission of the organization and will catch no one by surprise.

The intent of revealing physicians' performance to others is simple. Transparency of data drives physician behavioral change and lights a fire to utilize and implement proven tools to improve performance as measured by patient satisfaction.

STEP 7: USE MEASUREMENT TO DRIVE RESULTS

Tools and training for your physicians will be a continual process led by your Fire Starter. Measurement of patient satisfaction with progressive transparency of data will proceed as your organization matures. Next, data and tools must be used to drive results. Patient satisfaction percentile goals must be formally established and communicated within your organization. To truly impact physician behavior, individual physician compensation must, in some way, be impacted by patient satisfaction performance. The distribution of income based upon performance will need to be a medical group leadership decision. The following is an example of how it can be done.

Individual physician compensation model, utilizing national patient satisfaction percentile rank data:

Yearly or bi-annual bonus distribution:

- Above the 60th percentile nationally—Bonus received
- Above the 90th percentile nationally—Additional bonus received

- Below the 15th percentile nationally—Reduction in pay, unless enrolled in coaching or approved improvement program (see Chapter 8, Individual Physician Coaching)

STEP 8: CELEBRATE SUCCESS

High-performing physicians must be recognized as you roll out visibility and accountability for performance. Recognition for the individual physician is more important than many realize and ranks consistently as a principal predictor of physician satisfaction. Taking the time and making the effort to recognize and celebrate your best physicians accomplishes a number of important organizational goals, including:

- Recognizing and profiling excellence reinforces to everyone that high performance is an organizational priority.
- Recognition is known to replicate and duplicate the behaviors that earned the recognition.
- Recognition of physicians increases physician satisfaction and drives loyalty to the medical group.
- Profiling a group of high-performing physicians tends to "stir" the rank and file who inherently desire to be included amongst the best.

Strategies for recognition are numerous, and the methods selected are relegated to the medical group leadership. Options may include:

- Individual quarterly certificates, handed out and profiled at medical staff meetings for all those finishing the quarter in the 90th percentile and above, as measured by patient satisfaction.
- A physician award system, where several physicians who represent exemplary performance are selected per quarter, and are profiled amongst their colleagues.

- Personalized letters written by the medical director, sent to physicians' homes, simply thanking physicians for the extraordinary work that they do.
- A bi-annual physician excellence dinner, hosted by the medical leadership, where the top performing physicians are invited, dined, and thanked for the great work they have done.

STEP 9: DEAL WITH PERPETUAL LOW PERFORMANCE

As you measure patient satisfaction performance, you will find the same group of physicians will cluster at the bottom. As an organization committed to excellence, you must implement a strategic plan for these physicians. Three options exist. First, you do nothing and ignore them. This option will eventually impact your group's progress and is not a good option for the physicians, the group, or your patients. Second, you can fire them. Though this option unfortunately can become a necessity, it is expensive, it damages your reputation in the physician community, and it can negatively impact physician morale. Third, you can engage your physicians in individual coaching and mentoring, and make them accountable for their own improvement.

The fact is that communication techniques can be taught, and physicians can respond and improve given the tools and training. Chapter 3 (Physician Service Excellence Tools) and Chapter 8 (Individual Physician Coaching) review the tools and individual coaching approaches that work. The important element in your organization is to make a statement that sitting habitually at the bottom of the database in your group is not an option. Your medical group leadership will provide tools, training, and support to help physicians improve performance.

Driving physician performance and changing physician behaviors is a task that requires multiple forces working in coordination with each other. Core change efforts include a clear statement and commitment from physician leadership to service and operational excellence as a strategic priority. Next, the selection, training, and positioning of a physician "Fire Starter" to successfully champion the effort. Following this, a provision of tools, tactics, and training for physicians to drive the patient experience and the utilization of comparative ranking data to stir change. As the performance culture matures, the creation of specific performance standards to which physicians are held accountable. Along the entire process, a dedicated recognition of those who rise to the top and a helping hand to those who struggle.

The most important of all these organizational efforts is how the message of your commitment to excellence is imparted to your physician staff. It must be clear; it must be consistent; it must come from every tier of leadership. All efforts to improve physician performance will be deeply embedded in the simple commitment to provide extraordinary care to patients, to expand market share through patient testimony, and to harbor clinical excellence through collaboration, expertise, and trust.

Key Learning Points—Physician Implementation of Service Excellence

1. Physician leadership commits to service excellence as a core strategy for the medical group. Physician leadership must be willing to make an unwavering commitment to this effort and stand by this under all circumstances.

2. Select a physician Fire Starter. You will need a Champion who is respected in the group to lead this effort. The Fire Starter must be fully supported and trained to be effective.

3. Clearly define the role of your physician Fire Starter to support the goals of your organization.

4. Train your physician Fire Starter to lead.

5. Launch the commitment to excellence and train your physicians. Create a burning platform, create the case for service, define the physicians' central role in success, and provide physicians service tools that work to drive the patient experience.

6. Measure patient satisfaction and provide feedback. Provide physicians comparative data on their performance, with progressive performance transparency.

7. Use data results to drive performance. Begin to tie compensation to physician performance as your organization matures.

8. Celebrate success. Recognize your high performers.

9. Create a system to help low performers, and do not ignore physicians who struggle.

CHAPTER 8:

INDIVIDUAL PHYSICIAN COACHING

As your organization rolls out a commitment and vision for service excellence, and begins to provide prescriptive tools and leadership support to improve patient satisfaction, you will have physicians who fall below organizational standards. These will be physicians who think that they are doing things well in terms of how they treat patients, but the patient satisfaction numbers are just plain poor. You will find physicians are ambitious and competitive by nature, and the prospect of poor performance is unsettling to them, to say the least.

A required element of a commitment to service excellence for physicians is a mechanism to help individual physicians who need it. We have done extensive individual physician coaching and have found, almost uniformly, that physicians want help to get better, and often have little insight as to why patients say the things they say about them. It is incredibly disheartening for physicians to have those patients, who are the life blood of our business, say to us, "We don't think you are friendly; you don't explain things clearly; you didn't give me enough information; you didn't spend enough time with me; I don't have confidence in you; I wouldn't recommend you to my friends." That is the material translation of low patient satisfaction. For the good of the group, the good of the patients, and the long-term viability of the physician, tools must be deployed to get this fixed.

A process for individual physician coaching is a must-have for any organization that plans to move forward. A perpetual low-performing physician in your group interfaces with 20 patients daily, and each of those patients has the potential of telling 10 friends of their bad experience. A perpetual low-performing physician will "lead by example" a group of nurses and receptionists who will gravitate to the performance level of the physician. Low-performing physicians can have tremendous impact on the performance and reputation of your organization. Coaching intervention, done properly, can make physicians better.

IDENTIFYING PHYSICIANS FOR COACHING

The process of selecting which physicians will be coached is best left to hard data, as opposed to subjective leadership decisions. Analyzing data and making the decision to contact and intervene for a physician is best left to your medical director and physician Fire Starter, who are familiar with the coaching process.

The following data sets are best used to determine coaching candidates:

- Patient Satisfaction
  - Any physician below the 15th percentile nationwide on a quarterly basis should be considered a candidate for coaching.
  - The "cut off" number for your organization will be determined by the patient satisfaction tool used by your group, the performance of your physicians, and a consensus of your physician leadership.
- Patient Complaints
  - More than six complaints per year mandates coaching intervention.

- Peer Review
  - Physicians who are disrespectful and abrasive to colleagues should fall into disciplinary action, but often these physicians may benefit from coaching intervention as well.
  - "How to get along with colleagues in your medical group" can be prescriptive, teachable tools and should be used if physicians fall into this category.

As much as we like to rely on data to make coaching decisions, the subjective "call" of leadership will invariably come into play. Several supplemental points are helpful in selecting which physicians to coach.

- "Coachability" is a critical, subjective coaching criterium that calls for the judgment and experience of your physician leadership tasked with selecting physicians for coaching. You must determine who will be receptive to coaching, because almost no medical group has the time and resources to coach everyone who "qualifies."
- Newer physicians are traditionally "easier" to coach than well-established physicians. The general surgeon who has been in practice for 30 years who is called for coaching is less likely to change behaviors compared to the less established physician.
- A consistent trait of those who respond to coaching is the ability of the physician to gain insight to the fact that it is what they do that creates the patient perception of care. If the coached physician points a finger at staff, access, the measurement tool, or the parking conditions for low performance, and refuses to take any responsibility for their position, necessary behavioral change will not happen.

CONTACTING PHYSICIANS FOR COACHING

Once a decision is made to coach specific physicians, and a list of physicians is generated, you must contact your colleagues to let them know what will be happening. This can be awkward, but it is a very important part of the process to assure physicians understand exactly what is happening and why the coaching is being done. We suggest your physician Fire Starter or medical director make this initial contact. The physician is familiar with these leaders and will be more receptive to the coaching prospect. Given the content of the ensuing discussion, this is best done through appointment and done face to face.

Here is an example of what can be said to a physician who meets coaching criteria:

"Dr. Brown (Jim), I know you have been with the medical group for three years, and we are vested in your success here. Your quality and peer review have been excellent, but your patient satisfaction is not, and we want to help you. Our board of directors has required that physicians who score low in patient satisfaction get assistance. We have developed a coaching system that is designed to give you simple tools that will work. We have done this with many other physicians with good success. We will meet with you for one hour, review your patient satisfaction data, and give you tools to improve your patient satisfaction, based specifically on the patterns of what your patients are saying. We will then give you a summary of the recommendations and follow up to ensure you have the support to carry out this effort.

Jim, as you know, this group is now committed to performance, and patient satisfaction is one of our most important measures of success. This physician coaching is a requirement to get better and to help you succeed."

This conversation clearly explains the what and why of physician coaching. This contact needs to be made directly from a physician leader and not by letter or e-mail. This conversation also can be done by phone, but it is preferably done in person. If this effort is not positioned and communicated well at the outset, your physicians will feel very threatened and confused and will be less likely to come forward with receptiveness to change.

CONTENT OF COACHING

When we coach physicians, we deploy tools that are customized for that physician based on what the patients of that physician say. Most patient satisfaction tools will provide question-specific responses and rankings, allowing you to target which areas need work.

For example, if we see a "drop off" in patient satisfaction scores in response to the question, "Did your physician use language you could clearly understand?", we will provide specific tools for that question. We will go through mock clinical situations to see what the physician does now, and what it looks like to do it differently utilizing the trained tool. The specific tools we use are provided in Chapter 3 (Physician Service Excellence Tools).

In general, we never provide more than two specific tools for physicians during a training session. Which tools are selected depends on the pattern of responses from patients. What we find is that if physicians incorporate these tools into their practice, and commit to doing them for every patient, every time, nearly every element of a patient experience is positively impacted. For example, when you use tools that ensure patients have clear, simple explanations for diagnosis, treatment, or medications and physicians query for patient understanding, when patients are asked, "Did the physician use language you could understand?" or "Did the physician include you in decision making?" or even "Did the physician spend adequate time with you?", all of those questions are impacted by a single, effective tool that is consistently implemented.

Some organizations have used "shadowing" techniques, where coaches will actually go into the patient exam room with the physician and patient and observe a number of office visits. This is then followed by a "breakdown" of the visits and a write-up to summarize what is currently done and specific recommendations for changes.

WHO DOES THE COACHING

Many organizations will hire outside consultants to do this work. If this is done, we encourage partnership with a team of high-performing physician leaders who can assist in the selection and physician communication process. Individual physicians, including your physician Fire Starter, within your organization may also do the coaching. All coaches must be familiar and comfortable with the patient satisfaction tools, analysis of the data, and the specific tools we engage to change physician behavior and improve patient satisfaction.

COACHING FOLLOW-UP

We suggest tracking the performance of your coached physicians for at least one year. Information on service tools needs to be provided in written form to the coached physician within a week or two of the coaching. Results of patient satisfaction scores should be provided to physicians on a monthly basis so they can see the impact of their efforts. Monthly, brief phone follow-ups from the coach should be provided to ensure implementation remains consistent and questions and concerns are addressed.

Coaching physicians is a challenging and invigorating process. We have had physicians who come to us emotionally broken and on the brink of burnout. Frustrations seem to inherently arise for patients and physicians when patient needs are not met.

When physicians are given the tools, support, and guidance to provide better care and service to patients, patients treat physicians better. Physicians need to be recognized when they undertake and commit to change. They will find collaboration, enthusiasm, and making a difference begin to replace bitterness and cynicism. Again, it seems we best serve ourselves through our commitment to others.

Key Learning Points—Physician Coaching

1. In an organization that has committed to excellence, a commitment to help struggling physicians is a necessity.

2. Create standards for coaching intervention:

    a. Physicians <15th percentile in patient satisfaction for consecutive quarters

    b. More than six complaints per year

    c. Low peer review

    d. Physician must be "coachable."

3. Contacting physicians for coaching should be done personally, and the content of the conversation should include what is being done, why it is being done, and how it will be done.

4. The content of coaching is based on providing one or two service tools based upon "patterns" of patient responses in your patient satisfaction tool.

5. The key to improved results in coached physicians is consistent implementation of provided tools. Every patient, every time.

6. Provide follow-up to coached physicians with a written summary of behaviors to implement.

7. Provide coached physicians monthly patient satisfaction data to track response to efforts.

8. Provide coached physicians e-mail reminders on service efforts.

9. Recognize physicians who undergo change and who obtain results.

CHAPTER 9:

PHYSICIAN SELECTION

Great medical organizations are made up of great physicians. Great physicians can be made through cultivation, guidance, and training, which is a commitment worth every ounce of organizational resource and effort. Alternatively and additionally, great physicians can be selected. The selection of which physicians work for your organization can be one of the most important processes undertaken to ensure the talent and profile of physicians who will position your group for success. Clinical talent alone is no longer sufficient to drive the performance of your organization. The physician selection "toolkit" is a behavioral-based interview process that chooses physicians based on their communication skills, teamwork and collaboration, caring and compassion, judgment and problem solving, and leadership abilities.

Historically, the physician interview process is undertaken by physicians untrained in interviewing techniques, who frequently don't know what to ask, how to ask questions, and how to assess responses. Many of these critical physician hires are made on gut instincts, with little regard to asking the questions that predict, with reasonable certainty, the conduct of a prospective physician hire.

The purpose of instituting this process is to ensure consistency in physician selection and to populate your medical group with physicians who can position the organization for success.

Here are the steps in instituting behavioral-based interviewing for physician selection:

1. Select the physician interview team.
2. Create consensus on the physician requirements for your medical group.
3. Train physician interviewers.
4. Prepare for interviews.
5. Conduct interviews.
6. Make the selection.

SELECT THE PHYSICIAN INTERVIEW TEAM

The members of your interview team should include your medical director, department chairs, and other selected physicians. The physicians selected for the interview team must be those who have been identified as high-performing contributors to the medical group, who model the standards of the group in attitude and behavior as well as clinical competence.

Physician interview team members:

- Have a clear understanding of the physician job responsibilities
- Are willing to participate in training in behavior-based questioning and the peer interview process
- Communicate well and have strong listening skills

This team of interviewers will be responsible for all physician interviewing throughout the organization.

CREATE CONSENSUS ON THE PHYSICIAN REQUIREMENTS FOR YOUR MEDICAL GROUP

To ensure that this process works, the medical director, department chair, and physician interviewers must agree on the expectations of physicians who work for your medical group. What kind of physicians do you want to hire? The selected core behavioral competencies are specific predictors for physician success in the medical group setting.

By querying for experience and knowledge within each behavioral category, this selection process is designed to select physicians who treat staff, patients, and physician colleagues in a way consistent with the aspirations and mission of a medical group committed to clinical and service excellence.

The core behavioral competencies include:

- Teamwork and collaboration
- Caring and compassion
- Communication
- Judgment and problem solving
- Leadership

TRAIN PHYSICIAN INTERVIEWERS

Training physicians on *how* to interview is critical to success. Few physicians arrive with a competency in peer interviewing as a complement to their clinical experience, so it is important that interviewers are comfortable with this skill set. Designated, selected physicians who constitute the team of interviewers should understand the process and principles articulated in this chapter.

PREPARE FOR INTERVIEWS

1. Review the candidate's curriculum vitae and background.

2. Coordinate the interview.
   - Three physicians, including the medical director, the department chair of the department to which the applicant is applying, and a select member of the physician interview team

who will work in close proximity to the applicant physician will interview each applicant.

- Each team member will fill out the candidate evaluation form that includes a scoring matrix for applicant assessment.
- Each interviewer will ask five questions, including ONE from each of the behavioral competency questions provided (see Resource 2).
- Each interviewer will coordinate with other interviewers so that questions are not duplicated.

CONDUCT INTERVIEWS

1. Interviewers arrive on time. Applicants are evaluating you as much as you are evaluating them.
2. Interviewers should arrive with the candidate's CV, the list of questions to be asked, note paper, and the evaluation form.
3. Establish rapport with the candidate.
   a. Introduce yourself. Tell the candidate your position and how long you have been with the organization.
   b. Clarify and ask for professional information not included on the CV or any additional information on past experience.
   c. Make an effort to smile and make eye contact, and not to frown, cross your arms, or turn away from the candidate.
4. Ask your set of behavioral questions predetermined prior to the interview.
   a. As the candidate responds, score responses on a one to five scale, with five representing a response in which no further training or mentoring is required and an excellent match for the medical group.
   b. Take notes summarizing key points made by the candidate.

5. When asking questions, inquire about *specific* past job performance. Past actions are strong predictors of future performance.

   a. Use behavioral-based questions that explore how the applicant performed in real situations in the past so that you can evaluate how he or she will likely handle similar situations in your organization.

   b. This query approach is similar to one used by mortgage and credit card companies. Prospective creditors don't ask if applicants think it would be a good idea for them to pay their bills; they want to know if they have paid their bills in the past.

6. Clinical judgment and problem solving questions are not part of the behavioral-based format, but require the applicant physician to respond to a hypothetical clinical situation that helps assess the depth and experience of the candidate's clinical skills.

7. Questions should be open-ended. To determine what physicians have done in the past, use some of the following phrases:

   a. Tell me about a time when…

   b. Tell me exactly how you dealt with…

   c. Describe a situation…

8. With every question, probe for three elements we call the EAR:

   a. Event-The specific event

   b. Action-The action the applicant took

   c. Result-The result of the action

Continue to probe until you can elicit the three response components. Often an interviewer will need to prompt an applicant to complete an answer by asking, "And what happened then? What was the outcome?" Become comfortable with silence. These questions are difficult and will take applicants some time to respond.

9. Stay legal! Any question that is not related to the performance of the job itself leaves the organization vulnerable to legal action (see Resource 3 for questions you CANNOT ask).

10. Ask the candidate, "What questions do you have for me?" Strong candidates will know and have researched your organization and are likely to ask additional questions.

11. Close the interview graciously. You want to leave a good impression, whether or not the candidate is hired. Remember, the candidate will talk about your organization to colleagues and acquaintances.

12. Thank the candidate for meeting with you.

    a. Be sure your closing comments don't imply that you definitely plan to hire this specific person.

    b. Summarize the steps that will happen next and when the candidate will hear back from you.

13. Complete your evaluations of the candidate immediately. Make the recommendation while the interview is still fresh in your mind.

MAKE THE SELECTION

Selecting the physician hire from prospective candidates is the final step.

Steps in the final evaluation of the candidate:

1. Start with the completed evaluation form (Resource 1).

2. Provide a one to five score for each of the behavioral-based questions during the interview process.

3. Add the candidate's score, compute the average, and review notes.

4. Decide to "recommend" or "not recommend" and select the appropriate box.

5. As you evaluate the candidate, consider the following:

    a. Does this candidate match your culture?

    b. Are there areas of concern in a focused skill area that you need more information on?

    c. Are you evaluating based on specific examples of behavior?

    d. If there are areas of concern, can you train in these areas?

6. Never forget, do not compromise. Sometimes the best hire is the non-hire.

RESOURCE 1: SAMPLE INTERVIEW MATRIX TEMPLATE

Candidate _____

Position _____

Interviewer _____

Date _____

Core Competency Question (*Tell me about a time when you…*)	Score 1-5	Comments/Notes
1. TEAMWORK AND COLLABORATION		
2. CARING AND COMPASSION		
3. COMMUNICATION		
4. LEADERSHIP		
5. JUDGMENT AND PROBLEM SOLVING		
6. VALUE YOU WOULD BRING TO US		
TOTAL		
AVERAGE SCORE		

1:	2:	3:	4:	5:
-No experience	-Limited experience	-Specific experience	-Strong experience	-In-depth experience and
-No cited examples	-Few examples cited	-Specific cited examples	-Strong cited examples	ability to teach others
-Skills not evident	-Limited skills	-Evident skills	-Solid skills	-Exemplary cited examples
				-In-depth skills

Additional comments:

RECOMMEND [ ]   DO NOT RECOMMEND [ ]   107

RESOURCE 2: SAMPLE INTERVIEW QUESTIONS

Behavioral Category: Teamwork and Collaboration

1. Describe a situation in which you worked with a physician you didn't get along with. Tell me about that situation and how it worked out.
2. When you have been part of a group of physicians in the past, how did you determine whether the group was working well together? (Please give specific examples.)
3. Please describe a conflict you have had in the past with a fellow physician. How did you attempt to resolve the situation, and what is your relationship like now?
4. Tell me about your best practice situation with your colleagues in terms of how everyone worked together and what specifically made it the "best."
5. Describe a time when you felt you were getting the short end of the stick in a group setting with your physician colleagues and how you resolved the situation.
6. Tell me about a time when you were criticized by a physician colleague. How did you respond, and what was the outcome?
7. Tell me about a collaborative effort or project you have been a part of in your prior medical group or residency. What was your specific contribution?
8. Describe a time you had to address a staff member or nurse regarding a performance-related issue. What did you say or do and what happened?

Behavioral Category: Caring and Compassion

1. Tell me about a time when you went above the call of duty for a patient. What happened and what was the outcome?
2. Describe specific techniques you have used to convey and communicate that you care for patients and their clinical outcome.

3. What clinical situations have caused you the greatest frustration, and how did you deal with them? Please give specific examples.

4. Describe a time when you have had to deliver bad news to a patient and family. How did you specifically go about doing that, and what was the outcome?

5. Patient loyalty is key to a successful practice. Tell me what techniques you believe are important in creating patients who are loyal to you and the medical group. Please give examples of techniques you have used in the past.

Behavioral Category: Communication

1. Describe a time when you realized that you had to change a way in which you communicated to a staff member or fellow physician. What did you do, and what was the result?

2. Tell me about a time in which you realized that you had to change a way in which you were communicating to patients. What change did you make, and how did it work out?

3. If I talked to your prior receptionist/nurse, what would they say about you and how you conduct yourself with staff and patients?

4. "Word of mouth" can be an important marketing tool to medical practices. Tell me specifically how you have contributed in generating a positive patient word of mouth during your involvement in your previous medical practices.

5. Describe what you have done to create good first impressions with brand new patients.

6. Have you ever lost a nurse due to a personality conflict? Tell me what happened.

7. Have you ever left a position due to a personality conflict with leadership or a fellow physician? Please describe what happened.

Communication Knowledge Questions (Questions based on knowledge in a hypothetical situation, and not necessarily based on what they have done in the past)

1. Please describe how you would respond to this scenario: A patient calls for his PSA results on a Tuesday. He had his labs drawn a week previously. You request the chart to compare to prior levels, but you do not get the chart before leaving on vacation for two weeks. The chart and the PSA sit on your desk for two weeks until you return, when the patient was told he would be called within 24 hours with his results. What do you say to this angry patient when you realize what happened? The PSA is elevated, but no more so than the year prior.
2. A healthy 25-year-old female comes to your office and asks you to order a CA-125 blood test. Tell me how you proceed.
3. A previously healthy 58-year-old male comes to your office complaining of general fatigue and frequent urination. Laboratory evaluation reveals a blood glucose of 245, with no other abnormalities. You call the patient to review your findings. Tell me about your conversation.

Behavioral Category: Leadership

1. Tell me about a time you had to convince your physician colleagues to do something differently, and what you did to get that done. What were the results?
2. When you have had to lead change at your clinic site, how did you go about doing it? What was the outcome?
3. Tell me about an important goal you have set for yourself since residency and how you have gone about accomplishing it.
4. Describe a great physician mentor you have had in your past and what specifically made him or her great. Include the relationship you currently have with that person.

5. Tell me about a time when you have coached a member of your staff to improve his or her performance. What did you do? What were the results?

6. Tell me about a time when you motivated a group to do something. What method did you use, and why did you choose that approach? What was the result?

7. In the age of a nursing shortage, tell me what specifically you have done to keep your high-performing nurse.

8. Tell me about the best physician leader you have worked for. What specifically did that person do? What did you learn from him or her and how have you incorporated these skills into your personal leadership style?

9. Tell me about the work environment you have enjoyed most in the past. What did you like about it? How did you specifically contribute to this positive work environment?

Behavioral Category: Judgment and Problem Solving

1. Tell me about the busiest time you have ever experienced in a clinical work environment. How did you respond?

2. Tell me about a time that you have made a clinical mistake as the treating physician. What did you do, and how did it work out?

Judgment and Problem Solving Knowledge Questions
(Hypothetical situations, not eliciting applicant prior conduct)

1. While on call you receive a phone call at 10 p.m. from a nursing home where your colleague admits his patients. The nurse describes to you that one of your colleague's patients has developed shortness of breath over the past several hours. The patient is an 85-year-old male with a history of moderate dementia but no other known medical problems except for

hypertension. His oxygen saturation is 91 percent, his respiratory rate is 24, pulse is 100, and his temp is 99.0.

- Describe how you would work through this problem over the phone and what you would do next.

You learn that a call was placed to the daughter who has the DPOA for health care decisions, and she has requested that nothing be done and that only comfort measures be undertaken. You believe the patient has a treatable cause for his symptoms.

- How would you proceed?

2. You have 12 patients booked for a full morning. You are running on time and a 45-year-old male comes to your office with a chief complaint on your schedule as "heartburn." As you interview this patient, you realize that his "heartburn" is periodic non-exertional chest pressure. He has had no symptoms for the last 12 hours.

- How would you proceed?

3. You see a 39-year-old female for abdominal bloating, cramping, and dyspeptic symptoms of three weeks' duration. You diagnose a functional bowel condition and recommend over-the-counter symptomatic treatment. She returns in one week with similar symptoms, but denies fevers, nausea, vomiting, diarrhea, or weight loss. You provide her an empiric trial of a PPI and a fiber supplement. She tries this for a week and does not improve. She seeks a second opinion on her own. An abdominal/pelvic CT is done, which reveals probable metastatic ovarian CA. The patient changes physicians and is upset that you didn't make an earlier diagnosis.

- Tell me how you would have proceeded differently.

RESOURCE 3: QUESTIONS AN INTERVIEWER CANNOT ASK

DON'T ASK CANDIDATES:

- Age or anything that would indicate it, such as year of graduation
- Marital status or sexual preference
- Whether they have children or children's ages
- Whether they have ever filed for Worker's Compensation
- If they have ever been arrested
- Where they were born or live
- Whether they are a citizen
- How long they have lived in a particular location
- If they speak or write any other languages (unless job appropriate)
- If they have child care arrangements
- Whether they have a disability
- If they attend church or which one
- Any questions about religion, politics, or organizational affiliations
- What kind of car they drive, their credit or financial status
- What their maiden name is/was

PHYSICIAN SELECTION SUMMARY

Physician selection using behavioral-based interviewing creates selection consistency in two ways: by increasing physician ownership of the process and by enhancing the likelihood of hiring a candidate who fits the culture of your organization. Because past behavior is the best predictor of future performance, behavioral-based questions in peer interviewing generate specific responses to allow for greater confidence in selecting your physicians.

Having and selecting great physicians is the backbone of any medical group that succeeds. Instituting a selection process is critical to the long-term viability of your organization.

A complete copy of the Physician Selection Toolkit can be found at studergroup.com under "toolkits."

Key Learning Points—Physician Selection

1. Selecting the right physicians for your medical group is vital for long-term organizational success.

2. Behavioral-based peer interviewing is an interview technique that allows interviewers to ask questions and illicit responses that can predict the future conduct of physician applicants.

3. Select and train a team of physician interviewers who will conduct all interviewing for your organization.

4. Prepare for interviews by reviewing the applicant's CV and background information and select which behavioral questions each physician interviewer will ask.

5. Each interviewer will ask five questions and score responses on the scoring matrix (Resource 1).

6. Questions will be selected from a menu of questions (Resource 2) from each behavioral category, including caring and compassion, teamwork and collaboration, communication, judgment and problem solving, and leadership.

7. Interview evaluations will come with an average score on each of the questions, as well as a **recommend** or **do not recommend** for hire.

CHAPTER 10:

CREATING AND IMPLEMENTING PHYSICIAN BEHAVIORAL STANDARDS

Transformation of the culture of an organization requires the involvement of everyone. If standards of performance and standards of accountability are not equal within a workforce, a sense of resentment and unfairness will develop. When perceived imbalances of accountability and expectations persist, the sustainability of improvement that may have occurred will not be maintained, and an atmosphere of *why-do-I-have-to-do-it-if-they-don't?* will blossom.

The development of behavioral standards for physicians is essential for the implementation of service excellence for a medical group. In fact, one could say that it is difficult to implement any sense of standards of service, until the standards are clearly articulated. Do not assume that if you provide physicians the training and tools to drive the patient experience, that all of your physicians will actually do it. Creating standards of performance is the opportunity for your medical group physician leadership to create a platform for how your medical group will be run and how you will conduct yourselves. Standards simply say…this is how we do things here. Behavioral standards allow for consistency of service, so it no longer depends on which physician or which department, but is delivered by all physicians within all departments, all of the time. You cannot have some of your physicians returning patient phone calls on a timely basis and some not. You can't have some physicians returning pages promptly and some not. The medical group will never be able to establish a reputation of excellence with internal inconsistencies of performance. Creation and implementation of standards are fundamental to a cultural change for a medical group.

Perhaps even more important than delivering consistency of service and operations, articulated behavioral standards are a mechanism to deal with disruptive physicians more effectively and with greater authority. The American Medical Association has defined disruptive behavior as an interaction with physicians, hospital personnel, patients, family members, or others that interferes with patient care.[51] It is now clear in the medical literature that disruptive behavior by physicians impacts health care on nearly every front. Specific cited manifestations include upsetting patients and undermining patients' confidence in the care being received, upsetting staff enough so they refuse to work with a physician or delay calling when needed in fear of physician "wrath," delayed care through physician refusal to answer pages in a timely fashion, and the failure of staff to identify observed errors or quality issues due to physician intimidation.

In the 2004 American College of Physician Executives Survey, more than 95 percent of physician leaders encountered disruptive and potentially dangerous physician behaviors on a regular basis. In this survey, 70 percent of respondents reported that the same physicians are responsible for disruptive behaviors over and over again.

There is benefit in applying standards of behavior to all physicians proactively, as opposed to subjectively assessing "problem" physicians reactively based on nonstandardized assessments of conduct. Physician leaders despise dealing with difficult physicians and often wait far too long before disciplinary action is taken. In fact, the tipping point for intervention is often after something bad has already happened. A high-profile patient complaint or lawsuit, the departure of key staff members, or even patient harm arising from a dysfunctional work environment are all potentially irreversible consequences of ignoring a difficult physician.

The era of "that's just the way he or she is" is long gone, and now has evolved into institutional responsibility for workplace performance, cooperation, collegiality, respect, and accountability. The development of physician behavioral standards serves a core function of creating, communicating, and enforcing the operational and service platform of your medical group and is a necessity for behavioral consistency and the perception of fairness for everyone involved in the care of your patients.

CREATION OF PHYSICAN BEHAVIORAL STANDARDS

The process of developing physician standards will take work. The timing of the implementation of physician standards is important and should be done when your medical group physicians are "ready." Physicians need to see several things happen before they will graciously submit themselves to standards of conduct. If the timing is off, and the physicians are not sufficiently prepared for standards of performance, you will have a revolt on your hands. The timing and communication of the rollout can be as important as the content.

The following must be done prior to implementing physician behavioral standards:

- Physicians must see that the organizational commitment to excellence is a real, consistent, robust process that will serve them and the medical group well. Prior to launch, identify a major, chronic physician dissatisfier and fix it. Profile the solution to convey that the commitment to excellence will make their lives better. When physicians see that their voices are heard and action is taken, they will be more receptive to committing to organizational behavioral standards.

- Complete physician service training (see Chapter 7, Step 5) that includes the "elements" of your standards and their importance in driving patient satisfaction and medical group success. Physicians must see a very clear strategic reason why this must be done.
- Sufficiently communicate that these standards are coming and will be drafted by physicians, for physicians.
- When you begin to share with your physicians the emergence of Physician Behavioral Standards, share the following with them:
  - As an organization committed to being the best, certain disruptive physician behaviors will not be permissible.
  - Physician conduct is the foundation of the organizational commitment, and without consistent standards, progress will be limited.
  - Identify specific examples where the high variability of physician conduct undermines organizational efforts.
  - Communicate that disruptive physician behaviors will undermine workplace conditions, increase malpractice exposure, and compromise care to patients.
  - Remind physicians that they are the clinical workplace leaders. It is imperative that physicians consistently lead by example and model the behaviors consistent with the institutional commitment, and their conduct will set the standards for the organization.
- All physician leaders, with your Fire Starter at the point, must stand strongly behind this and be willing to defend it...*this is the right thing to do for the patients and the right thing to do for the group, and if we want to be the best and establish a reputation of excellence, all of us must commit to these standards...*

- Determine how these standards of conduct will be enforced prior to release. This is often the most difficult leadership decision. We suggest that clear, egregious violations of the standards of conduct for your medical group be met with formal disciplinary action according to medical group policy and bylaws. To be effective, these standards must have some teeth.
- The policy for these standards must be clear. Formal disciplinary processes must be engaged should repeated violations of your standards of conduct arise. (We suggest that **repeated** violations engage these disciplinary processes.) Even the best of physicians can have a single lapse of judgment.
- The elements of standards of conduct should be drafted by a group of respected leadership physicians so that consensus is obtained from a variety of physicians from a variety of specialties.

DETERMINING ELEMENTS OF PHYSICIAN BEHAVIORAL STANDARDS

Which behaviors you will include in physician behavioral standards will ultimately be at the discretion of the physician leadership of your organization. In fact, there are some groups who simply use the same general behavior standards for all staff, nurses, and physicians throughout the entire organization. We believe that there is an opportunity to address specific physician behaviors and responsibilities that can be aligned to meet the performance aspirations of your group that don't necessarily apply to other clinical positions.

Here is a list of physician behaviors that a group may place under consideration for institutional implementation:

- Return patient phone calls on the day the call was placed.
- Return pages in a timely fashion.
- Work cooperatively and respectfully with staff and nurses for the good of patient care.
- Arrive to work on time.
- Submit charges for services provided in a timely fashion.
- Never use language with any member of the health care team that is belittling and diminishes an individual's sense of worth within the organization.
- Never criticize another physician's treatment or actions in the presence of staff or patients.
- Interact and communicate with physician colleagues in a respectful, cooperative way for the good of patient care.
- Conduct yourself with patients in a manner that fosters patient satisfaction and loyalty to our medical group.

These are simple references to operational and service issues that align physician behavior with what is good for the organization and the patient.

In creating your medical group physician behavioral standards, consider the following:

- The more general you describe the desired conduct, the easier it is to monitor, implement, and gain physician support.
- We discourage including clinical competence within these standards. Quality and peer review processes should deal with this, and a behavioral contract is not the place to stipulate clinical competence.
- Instituiton of physician behavioral standards should occur during new physician orientation and contracting. Hiring and orientation are critical opportunities to clearly state what your medical group stands for and what is expected of physicians.

Even with a well-constructed and communicated plan for physician standards rollout, you may still have a minority of physicians protest your new behavioral standards. The groups at greatest risk for physician protest are the groups who have had long, distinguished histories of success doing things just as they always have. Having recently rolled out these standards, there is a repetition of concerns and questions that come from a small, but frequently vocal group of physicians.

Here is a list of physician concerns frequently heard in response to behavioral standards rollout:

- If most of us are doing most of these things, why is it that all of us have to participate in this?

ANSWER: In most groups, most physicians do a reasonable job with the core behaviors referenced in most codes of conduct. The reason for enforcing this for every physician is that it articulates and demands standards that the group cannot deviate from. Confronting low-performing, disruptive physicians becomes infinitely easier when all medical group physicians have signed and committed to clear organizational standards. By standardizing expectations of conduct, it also standardizes when violations of expectations occur, making for much more efficient, timely intervention. Traditionally, in the absence of standards, the intervention for a difficult physician is delayed, often after notable damage is done to the reputation of the medical group.

- We seem to be doing fine without these standards. Why do we have to do this now?

ANSWER: Even a single physician, seeing 25 patients a day, interfacing daily with numerous staff, receptionists, and nurses throughout the organization, who violates the organizational code of conduct, can undermine the great work of 10 of his conscientious, diligent colleagues. If your group has a number of "low performer" physicians, your group will never establish a reputation of excellence in the community, or even within your own organization. Reports about negative experiences, whether they be from patients or support staff, disseminate in much greater numbers and with much greater vigor than those about positive experiences. The medical marketplace has changed radically, and patients are now active, intelligent consumers who shop with their feet. Being "good" is not good enough in health care. To earn lifelong patient loyalty, to drive word of mouth referrals, to attract and retain the best staff, to rise above the competition, and to establish a reputation of excellence, you must be great. You must be great all of the time. These standards are core operational and service competencies that great organizations must do without exception.

- What is this, the Boy Scouts? I'm a physician; why do I have to sign this?

ANSWER: Occasionally physicians, particularly ones who have been successful doing things the right way for many years, can be taken aback being asked to sign something so obvious. Take this as an opportunity to position them well. Let them know that you are keenly aware of the fact that we have built the success of this practice on great physicians, like them, doing the right thing for patients and the right thing for staff. And let them know that as we have grown as a medical group, it is essential to create and communicate a standard of conduct that assures we never compromise the standards that built this group. If necessary, provide them information and evidence regarding groupwide inconsistency in group conduct. This is so important that nothing can be left to chance. Ask them for their support as a respected physician colleague.

- What are you going to do if I don't sign these standards?

ANSWER: This is the issue that will challenge your physician leadership more than any other and there is not an easy answer to this question. Consider the following in deciding the best response to this situation, which will most certainly arise.

- It is not so much whether they sign or don't sign a behavioral standard; it is whether they conduct themselves in a way that supports the mission and values of the medical group and is consistent with physician standards throughout the organization.
- The "non-negotiable" element of physician behavioral standards is the integrity of the standards themselves. Clear, repeated violations of stated standards must engage a response—otherwise, you have no standards. You may choose not to force the signature of a high-performing physician, who, for whatever reason, refuses to sign this code of conduct, but always and consistently does things in a way that fulfills the mission of the group. This situation is not a battle worth the division it can create.
- If a low-performing physician refuses to sign the code of conduct, engage a disciplinary process based on performance, not whether the physician signed or didn't sign the contract.
- Be prepared to hear protest on this issue. If you make decisions based on clearly communicated standards of conduct that are a necessity to medical group performance and individual physician success, we anticipate you will meet little resistance.

Key Learning Points—The Development and Implementation of Physician Behavioral Standards

1. The development and implementation of physician behavioral standards are a necessity for consistent, predictable performance from physicians.
2. Standards for physicians will convey to the rest of the organization that everyone is "on board" and everyone is accountable to the organizational mission.
3. To launch physician standards effectively:
   a. Demonstrate that your journey to excellence will make physicians' practices better, making them more receptive to do their part.
   b. Train your physicians, which should include the components of behavioral standards as precursors to organizational success.
   c. Keep physicians informed as to why, when, and how the standards will roll out.
   d. Remind physicians that they are the workplace leaders and their conduct will determine the standards of the organization, thus the articulation and adherence to standards becomes imperative.
   e. Inform physicians that the standards will be created by physicians, for physicians.
   f. Stand strong with unified leadership that this is the right thing to do for the group, the patients, and the physicians.
   g. Determine the "consequences" for violation and communicate this to physicians prior to the launch.
4. Determine the components of your standards, seeking physician behaviors that align physician conduct with your organizational mission.
5. Assemble a team of respected physicians within the medical group tasked with the creation of group-wide standards.

CHAPTER 11:

PHYSICIAN BEST PRACTICES

Best practices are service and operational initiatives that make physician practices exceptional. When best practices are encountered by patients, they make an impression, they define excellence, they are above expectations, and will consistently create loyalty and word of mouth marketing. We will provide a list of efforts that have been developed and implemented at our institution.

THE PATIENT AGENDA

The patient agenda is a simple document that serves the patient's desire to be "heard." The patient agenda allows the patient's concerns and questions to drive the visit, and creates clear objectives for the encounter.

HOW IT WORKS:

As patients come in for routine, scheduled appointments with their physicians, they are given a form by the receptionist. The receptionist, using scripted keywords, says to patients:

"Dr. Beeson would like to have you fill out this form to be sure all of your concerns are addressed during your visit. Write down the questions or issues that are most important to you and Dr. Beeson will cover those concerns with you."

The patient agenda serves a number of important objectives:

- Occupies patients while they're waiting to be seen
- Is a proactive inquiry for patients to let them know this visit will be on their terms, and driven by their concerns and questions
- Improves the time efficiency of an office visit by preventing the physician from having to "fish" for the true reason for the appointment
- Prevents the dreaded doorknob phenomenon, where potentially serious and time-consuming issues blind-side physicians at the end of the visit

A practice that is committed to meeting the needs of its patients is a practice that will thrive and grow. Creating a means to construct all visits to ensure that patients have the opportunity to clearly state what it is that they want from the visit is a requisite to meeting those patient needs. The patient agenda is a best practice that is fundamental for organizations committed to providing patient-centered care.

Please see the sample patient agenda used in some of our clinics:

Welcome to Sharp Rees-Stealy Medical Group. Our goal is to provide you exceptional medical care and to be sure that all of your health concerns are addressed during your visit with Dr. Beeson. Take a moment to write down questions or issues you would like to cover with the doctor during your visit today.

1._____

2._____

3._____

Please check the other items that apply to this visit:

☐ **Medication Refills**

List medications you need refilled, along with the doses and how often you take them.

_____

_____

_____

_____

☐ **I need forms filled out.**

Please fill out your portion of the form prior to your visit and state the type of form you have (sports physical, DMV Exam, etc.).

_____

PHYSICIAN CALLBACKS

The physician callback may be the single most powerful tool physicians can use to grow their practice, earn patient loyalty, and develop a reputation of excellence in the community. Physician callbacks in the outpatient setting is an unsolicited call from a physician to follow up with a patient seen a day or two before.

HOW IT WORKS:

Throughout the course of a day, a physician will see a variety of patients, some of which come in for acute illnesses. At the discretion of the physician, some of these sick patients will be "tagged" for next day callbacks. On the following day, the treating physician will call these patients to check on their clinical status.

The physician callback would go something like this:

A patient is seen for acute bronchitis with secondary bronchospasm and wheezing. The physician prescribes an antibiotic and a steroid taper as well as a bronchodilator. A day or two following the visit, the physician, referring to his callback sheet, calls the patient and says:

Physician: Hello, John. This is Dr. Beeson calling. I'm checking in to see how you're feeling.

Patient: Dr. Beeson? You have got to be kidding me! I am beginning to feel better, thank you.

Physician: Do you have any questions about the medications that I had prescribed for your bronchitis?

Patient: No, they are working well.

Physician: Excellent. Call me if there is anything else you need.

Patient: I will. Thanks again, doc.

Having done hundreds of these calls, this is how 90 percent of them go. The average duration is between 90 and 120 seconds. Occasionally there is a question on a medication, or a side effect issue, but the majority of patients are delighted and amazed that you have called. A patient who receives this call will never leave you and will tell five to ten people about what you did.

More importantly, you can find out critical clinical information that allows you to modify treatment.

Not long ago I admitted an elderly patient to the hospital for community-acquired pneumonia. We treated her with IV antibiotics and she improved after just a day and a half in the hospital. I discharged her home. I called her the day following discharge as part of the callback effort. "I don't feel as well as I did when I left the hospital," she told me. I had her come to the office. Her fever had returned, the white count had climbed, and her condition had clearly worsened. I changed her therapy, saw her back the next day, and she ended up doing well. The callback prevented a more serious clinical outcome.

The next day the patient said to me, "You must love what you do to call me at home like you did. You are the best doctor I have ever had in my 85 years." I now take care of her husband, her extended family, and her entire block.

Here is a sample form of the physician callbacks we use in our clinic:

Patient	MRN	Date of Visit	Condition	Date of Call	Follow-up
John Jones	12-33-45	1/9/06	Asthma flare	1/11/06	Improved

The physician callbacks are a powerful marketing and clinical tool. If done consistently, they will grow your practice and improve the quality of care provided. For new physicians starting a practice, or groups seeking increased market share, hardwiring this initiative will create significant return on investment through patient loyalty and word of mouth referrals.

THE PHYSICIAN CODE

A physician code is a document that profiles how the physicians in your medical group treat patients, staff, and each other. The physician code can be an effective physician orientation tool for new physicians to communicate a clear outline in terms of the values and behaviors that drive your organization. The physician code is also effective as a platform for physician training as you engage physicians in the prescriptive necessities to cultural and behavioral change. The specific content of your physician code will be determined by your physician leadership, but an example of our physician code is provided here as a guide.

Here is what the physician code looks like in our organization:

SHARP
REES-STEALY
MEDICAL GROUP

PHYSICIAN CODE

The Mission of Sharp Rees-Stealy Medical Group is to improve the health of our community through a caring partnership with patients, physicians, and employees. Our goal is to offer quality services that set community standards and exceed expectations in a caring, convenient, affordable, and accessible manner.

The ability of the medical group to successfully fulfill our Mission is dependent on physicians. Each of us is a leader within our sphere of influence and how we treat patients, colleagues, and staff will set the tone for how care is delivered. We can expect better from those around us only when we do better ourselves and lead by example.

We seek to create ideals that define the type of physician who works for Sharp Rees-Stealy. Most importantly, we seek to provide an atmosphere to help physicians flourish professionally and personally, and to create a group that is defined by providing exceptional care to its patients, staff, and fellow physicians.

RELATIONSHIP TO STAFF

We will:
• Treat staff with dignity and respect.

- Work to lead a team where our philosophy, integrity, commitment, compassion, and caring is observed by those around us.
- Strive to make others better by expecting more of ourselves.
- Influence and communicate with those around us in a positive and cooperative way.
- Thank and recognize those who allow us to do what we do.
- Look for opportunities to do things better.
- Listen to the input of others and take an active ownership role to implement change.
- Educate rather than criticize.
- Work to be leaders who are respected because of our actions.

RELATIONSHIP TO PHYSICIANS

We will:
- Treat our colleagues with respect.
- Communicate effectively with each other to enhance continuity and quality of care.
- Look for the good in others and share these views with patients to improve perception and experience with Sharp Rees-Stealy primary and specialty care physicians.
- Foster the spirit of teaching and learning from each other.
- Look for opportunities to make each other better.
- Never criticize another physician's treatment or actions amongst staff or patients, but view differences as opportunities to improve.
- Encourage fun and interaction amongst colleagues both in and out of the workplace.
- Honor the uniqueness of others.
- Treat our colleagues in the way in which we want to be treated.
- Give a helping hand should someone need it.

RELATIONSHIP TO PATIENTS

We will:
- Treat patients with respect and dignity.
- Learn about the person as well as the condition.
- Work together with our patients as a team.
- Strive to make each patient feel as though he or she is our only patient.
- Make patients feel that we are always on their side because effective care can never be delivered in opposition.
- Engage, listen, and clearly explain issues to our patients so that time spent with us exceeds their expectations.
- Aim to return phone calls promptly.
- Thank patients for waiting if we are running late.
- Earn patients' loyalty through our behavior.

The Task of Medicine…
Cure sometimes, relieve often, and care always…

Perhaps the most powerful application of this kind of behavioral code is to place it where it can be seen by patients. Placing your physician code in the exam rooms of your facility, signed at the bottom by the physicians, is a powerful and highly visible communication of your commitment. Nearly all patients, as they wait to see the physician, will read the commitment your physicians have made. More importantly, the mere presence and visibility of specific standards of conduct create physician accountability for behaviors articulated in the code. If your code states that physicians will thank patients for waiting should they be running late, what will physicians do when entering an exam room where that is written on the wall, signed by them?

RECOVERY CARD

Even in the best of clinics, circumstances arise where the medical group falls short of patient expectations. The medical group response to these service shortfalls can define the patient experience and perception of your organization. Remember, the well-executed service recovery drives higher patient satisfaction than if nothing had gone wrong in the first place. The service recovery card is a simple way for receptionists, nurses, and physicians to implement and execute recovery at the frontline, whenever and every time it happens.

HOW IT WORKS:

The following scenarios seem to be the most common service shortfalls that occur in the outpatient arena:

- Excessive waits in the reception area (usually greater than 30 minutes after the scheduled appointment time).
- Not returning calls to the patient on the day we said we would.
- Patients returning to pick up prescriptions or forms, and they were not completed.
- Not providing diagnostic testing information to patients when indicated.

When these situations arise, service recovery as outlined in Chapter 5 should be engaged. Following this "on-site" recovery, we send a follow-up service recovery card. It is signed by those involved in the care of the patient, especially the physician and nurse, regardless of who was to "blame."

The card looks something like this:

Dear Mr. Jones,

We want to apologize for the excessive wait that occurred during your visit with us on August 14th.

The goal of the Sharp Rees-Stealy Medical Group is to provide you exceptional customer service, in addition to the best medical care. We look forward to providing you better service during your next visit with us, and please feel free to contact us if you have any questions or comments.

Kindest Regards,
Stephen Beeson, MD (signed)
Francesca Funk, LVN (signed)
Nina Chinualt, RN, Site Manager (signed)

It is very important that the recovery card be specific to the patient and to the situation; otherwise it becomes "generic" with little value or sincerity. We recommend that the card be signed by leadership, showing the patient that this problem is important to us and made its way to those who manage the organization.

The most important process for effective service recovery is to train your staff to know when it happens. It should be expected for them to report when service falls short and they should be empowered with the tools and training to effectively recover. A letter signed by the nurse, manager, and treating physician regarding service shortfalls will exceed patient expectations. More importantly, having a specific process that must be engaged when shortfalls occur will make the staff and physician more aware and vigilant with the operational performance standards of your organization and can reduce the necessity of recovery.

CHAPTER 12:

PHYSICIAN SATISFACTION IN THE AGE OF EXCELLENCE

Committed, passionate physicians will make everyone around them better. They will create loyalty and dedication of their staff and will have patients who market their practice to the highest level. These are the physicians who are the foundation of a reputation of excellence and are the cornerstone to the success of a medical group.

What are the clinical work conditions that help physicians become exceptional and an inspiration to others? Why is it that other physicians become so negative about what they do that they seem to undermine organizational efforts through endless cynicism, poisoning the spirit of everyone around them?

It is important to understand that physician satisfaction is a requisite for physician receptiveness for the work that needs to be done to make your organization great. When physicians are frustrated with leadership responsiveness and operational issues, getting them to engage service efforts becomes significantly more difficult. Concurrent to physicians' engagement efforts must be a tangible demonstration that your organization is equally committed to physicians. It is not necessary to "fix" all that troubles physicians prior to physician engagement, but it is important to have an environment where physicians' voices are heard and visible action is taken on their input.

Additionally, physician satisfaction impacts clinical quality, patient satisfaction, physician turnover,[52] physician well-being,[53] and productivity. Establishing an environment that allows the workhorse of your organization to thrive is a necessity to all organizational aspirations.

Predictors and drivers of physician satisfaction are not complex and are consistently observed in the literature. We will provide an outline of what physicians need to observe and experience within your organization to increase the probability of full collaboration with your organizational efforts. What may be most important to realize is that the pathway to physician satisfaction is to focus our efforts on physician engagement. Physician engagement is a means to address the leading dissatisfier in the physician workplace, which is the loss of physician autonomy and the ability to have an impact on practice operations. Physician involvement, participation, and leadership will drive greater operational performance and, more importantly, will foster ownership, influence, and fulfillment as physicians lead efforts for change.

WHAT PHYSICIANS NEED:

1. Quality
A clear commitment to clinical excellence is imperative to physician engagement. Clinical quality measures and initiatives to support outcomes must be profiled as critical items for your group. Nearly all physicians are inherently committed to quality efforts, and it should never be perceived that service and operational efforts are "replacing" clinical priorities.

2. Physician Input
Eliciting input from physicians is the means to have physicians' voices heard. Physicians having a say in practice operations and control over what they do consistently ranks as most important to physician satisfaction. Several strategies are effective in soliciting physician input regarding clinical operations.

- **Survey your physicians.** Internal surveys can be developed to determine what is going well and what needs improvement. Your physician survey should occur on an annual basis.
- **Encourage physician participation in clinic operations.** Physician representation is needed in clinical site operations and service efforts. The buy-in and support for organizational efforts is much greater when physicians actively participate and "own" efforts within a clinical site.

Consider a monthly meeting for a clinic site involving physician and administrative leadership for the purpose of planning service and operational efforts. The agenda of these meetings should include:

- Clinic site performance objectives, including:
    - Service (patient satisfaction)
    - People (employee and physician satisfaction)
    - Finance (copay collections, revenue targets, etc.)
    - Quality (clinical quality measures)
    - Growth (growth targets, disenrollment rates, etc.)
- Setting specific performance objectives under each performance measure ("Pillar").
- Creating action items with specific timelines for each objective.
- Assigning leadership accountability for each action item as well as follow-up to be reported to the committee.

Here is an example of a site meeting agenda designed to drive operational and service performance:

StuderGroup®	Clinic Site Physician and Administrative "Site Excellence" Leadership Meeting September 1, 2006	Attendees:
Pillar	**SITE PERFORMANCE OBJECTIVES AND CURRENT STATUS**	**Action Items-Date**
Service	Goal: Patient Satisfaction at the 90th percentile Current: Patient Satisfaction at the 73rd percentile	Staff-Develop process to inform all patients of waits if over 15 minutes. Implement by 11/1/06 Nursing-Keywords "for your comfort" with all patients during check-in. Implement by 10/1/06 MDs-Return patient calls on same day by 6 pm. Implement by 10/1/06
People	Goal: Nursing turnover reduction to 8 percent Current: Nursing turnover is 14 percent	Institute 30 and 90-day follow-up meetings with supervisors for all new hires. Implement by 12/1/06
Finance	Goal: Co-pay collection to 98 percent Current: Co-pay collection is at 90 percent	Institute process where co-pay collection integrates with the check-in process. Present new process at 10/1 meeting for review. Implement by 11/1/06
Quality	Goal: All patients assessed for tobacco use history Current: Chart audit-42 percent of all patients were asked about a smoking history	Include a standard tobacco use question to be completed after vital signs obtained. Implement by 12/1/06
Growth	Goal: 4 percent growth per year Current: Enrollment at 1 percent growth for the year	New physicians to speak at senior center (Dr, Jones and Smith) with an audience of 200 seniors Track disenrollment by physician. Present at 10/1 meeting Physician Modular Training- on "Creating patient loyalty." Complete by 12/1/06

The input of physicians on service and operational measures will drive accountability and execution of the administrative team. When physicians participate in specific performance action items, hitting objectives grows more probable. If service and operational objectives are rolled out without the input and leadership of physicians, the physicians will not "own" them and will be less vested in ensuring their success.

3. Organizational Responsiveness

Data collected from your physician satisfaction survey can lay the foundation and priority list for physician concerns. Medical groups that have high physician satisfaction are ones that have elicited the opinions of their physicians on the operations of the group and that have created ways to swiftly address dissatisfiers and profile solutions to physicians. From your collected data, a visible strategic response is critical. The organizational leadership should assemble administrative and physician leaders who are accountable for physician satisfaction survey solutions. A timely response to a physician dissatisfier is very important in proving to physician skeptics that this "commitment to excellence" is indeed something that will make their lives better. "You asked; we responded!" must be conveyed to physicians in a systematic way. When physicians articulate what it is they need, and nothing is done, the credibility of the leadership is compromised.

Organizational responsiveness can create leverage for the organization when physicians are asked to step up and lead. When physicians witness that this process is a credible transformation that yields observable changes in practice operations, physician resistance will fade. Organizational response improves workplace satisfaction and physicians are more likely to do what is asked of them to support the organizational mission.

4. **Reward and Recognition**

   Physician professional fulfillment correlates highly with recognition physicians receive for the work that they do. Never underestimate how important physician recognition is in sustaining physicians in an intrinsically demanding profession. Reward frequently and visibly, and align rewards with desired behaviors.

   It is rare for a medical group to develop processes to recognize physicians, but this should be considered a must-have in terms of driving physician satisfaction and engagement. Here are suggestions on how this can be done:

   • On a quarterly basis, draft a personally written and signed letter from your medical director to be sent to the homes of all physicians who finish in the top 15 percent nationwide for patient satisfaction.

   • Nursing and administrative leadership should send thank you notes to physicians, specifically recognizing those who have demonstrated leadership and participation in the clinic's efforts, or who model behaviors consistent with service excellence.

   • Create awards for physicians where physicians can submit nominations for colleagues profiling extraordinary care. The award recipients are announced at staff meetings where the story is told and winners are recognized amongst their physician colleagues.

   • At staff meetings, take a moment to recognize new physicians in the group, those who have participated in public service efforts, and those who have done something personally that would warrant recognition by colleagues.

The benefit of developing a reward and recognition culture for physicians is several-fold.

Physician reward and recognition will:

- Improve physician satisfaction by recognizing and appreciating physician work.
- By profiling what it is that captures recognition, leadership is making a statement that providing extraordinary care is a medical group priority.
- Recreates and reinforces the recognized behavior.
- Provides guidance and examples to other physicians as to what it is that defines exceptional clinical experiences by telling the stories of the physician award recipients.

5. Collaboration

The collaborative clinic work environment is stimulating and can be fun, even in the midst of an intense schedule. The relationship with your nurse and support staff needs to be cooperative, supportive, and collaborative where the team works together for the good of the patient. Create a work environment where people smile, laugh, help one another, and have fun together doing demanding, purposeful work. Physicians and staff can spend as much time at the office as they do at home, and the dynamics of those relationships can have a strong influence on the color of the day.

So how does one foster a collaborative, supportive work environment? Here are some suggestions:

- Get to know your staff. Know them by name, and ask them questions such that you get to know them as people as well as employees. Building relationships with those you work with all day, every day will improve work conditions for the staff and the physician.

- Plan events for your staff and their families. Every summer our clinic site will have a pool party at my house, where we all swim and barbeque. We talk about the funny things that happen that day for months afterwards. Shared experiences and history together will drive the staff's ability to be loyal to you, the organization, and the patients you treat together.
- Thank your staff for what they do. If your nurse has performed well throughout a busy day, thank her for doing a great job. A few attentive words can make the toughest of work conditions rewarding.

The relationships with those we spend all day with have a significant impact on the physician and staff work experience. Staff stay and leave based upon the relationships they create, and not necessarily the conditions or pay in the workplace. We retain staff and sustain physicians through a respectful, collaborative, purposeful work experience, dedicated to making a difference for patients.

6. **Collegiality**

The relationships that physicians in your group have with each other may be the most important single factor to protect against physician burnout. Physicians who feel isolated, alone, and even belittled will fade quickly in the rigors of a daily practice. A disrespectful work environment will decrease physician satisfaction and will drive physician turnover. An environment that promotes helpfulness, cooperation, respect, and a willingness to help a colleague in need will improve the performance of your physicians. Collegiality and friendships among colleagues is consistently ranked as one of the most important predictors of the medical group physician experience.

How do you develop a group that creates collegiality amongst its physicians?

- Develop a zero tolerance policy for disrespectful communication amongst physicians, and be willing to stand by this.
- Develop physician behavioral standards that include how physicians in your group treat colleagues.
- Train your physicians to "manage up" and to position colleagues well in the eyes of patients.
- Assign new physicians to your group a physician mentor. A mentor is an experienced physician who can answer questions and provide guidance as new physicians orient to the new practice.
- Create opportunities for physicians to interact socially. Our medical group has several events per year, including two all-physician dinner dances, a tennis tournament, and an annual CME retreat attended by approximately 100 of our physicians and their families.

Groups that succeed are groups that are built not only on a commitment to service and operational excellence, but are built on physician relationships, camaraderie, and friendships. In order for a group to stand firmly on a platform of excellence, and to successfully embark on a challenging organizational journey to be the best, the members of your team must respect each other, cooperate with each other, and help each other.

7. **Money**

Money is a strong determinant of physician satisfaction. The reason we address this for physicians is to reveal the context of income to other predictors of physician satisfaction. Many of us have known colleagues who have left good practices with good medical groups, for the "big money" usually offered in a far away place. When they arrive, they are often dumped on by "colleagues," screamed at by patients waiting impatiently to see the long-awaited replacement physician, and beaten up by brutal call schedules. They wonder why in the world they ever left. Money is important, but money in the absence of a respectful, collaborative work environment with a medical group committed to doing the right thing for the patient and physician can quickly lose its luster.

Additionally, epidemiological data suggests that true happiness appears more related to personality factors such as high self-esteem and feelings of personal control and appears to be unrelated to the ownership of consumer goods.[54]

8. **Physician Satisfaction through Our Commitment to Excellence**

Quality, efficiency, physician input, organizational responsiveness, reward and recognition, collegiality, collaboration, and competitive income will create an environment for physician longevity. But what is it that defines the exceptional physician career? To what degree is our professional destiny determined by the environment created for us, and to what degree is our fulfillment a function of our response to conditions around us?

Five years ago I found a single day's work physically, intellectually, and emotionally exhausting. Patients' long lists of complaints began to frustrate and drain me, interfering with my ability to get out of the clinic and home to my family. I saw every patient added to my schedule as an additional burden to me, and every patient call a tiresome task. I had difficulty connecting with patients, and found myself having less and less to give. The less I committed myself to the patient interaction, the more distant I became from those entrusting me with their care. I was 36 years old and burning out, not enjoying what I had spent most of my life to achieve. I became further disillusioned by the fact that many of the patients I was seeing occupied my time with self-limited disease, leaving me little opportunity to treat and cure, which was my benchmark for success and the principle reason I pursued this profession.

What happened? I lost my edge, lost my focus, and lost my love for what I do. I spent some time trying to grab an elusive flame that I knew I once had. I thought about what it was that kept my head up through residency and the first seven years of my practice.

In time, I found it again on my own. It came to me as clear as day, as I finished a visit in which I thought I had done little for a patient that I knew didn't need to see me. A mother had called me to thank me for seeing her son earlier in the day for a sore throat. He didn't have strep, but I cultured him to make them feel like I had done something. I spoke with this high school boy who happened to be going to the same high school I had graduated from 20 years earlier. He had questions about medicine as a career choice, and we spent the majority of our time recreating the vigors and adventures of a medical education passage. I enjoyed our brief exchange, but frankly forgot about it as I waded through my patients, waiting for a clinical find to pique my interest. The mother who called me didn't thank me for swabbing the young man's throat. She called me to thank me for rescuing her son. He too had lost his way, and struggled with depression, loneliness, and finding something of purpose in his life. The mother told me how difficult it had become for her to watch her bright young son lose interest in all that he had. The mother told me that after his visit he had awakened with a renewed passion, enthusiasm, and interest for something that she hadn't seen in years. She felt as though her son had returned, and she thanked me for making a difference.

Things changed for me quickly, as I began to see patients differently. Patients were now an opportunity to help, to make things better. I committed to seeing every patient through these eyes, and refused to let cynicism and resentment spoil my touch. I no longer relied on a cure to define my success, but cultivated caring, trust, and partnership, which I could do every time.

My practice grew, compliments soared, and complaints were zero. At the end of 2005, my patient satisfaction finished in the 99th percentile in the national database, and I was seeing more patients per day than I ever had. Multiple calls would come to me daily requesting an exception to my closed practice, and I received a nomination as one of the Top Doctors in San Diego for 2005 and 2006 by *San Diego Magazine*.

I found patients responded to my efforts by becoming better patients. Patients thanked me for what I was doing for them. The best medical care, which I had solely relied on to sustain me, was now coupled with a patient relationship founded on partnership and trust. Medicine became fun again, as I became vested and fed by making an impact and making lives better. The emotional return for me sustained my change such that I would never go back to the place I had been before. I grabbed what I had lost, and rekindled the spirit of what medicine can do.

So we talk of physician satisfaction. Is it the workload, money, and autonomy that we hear over and over again? Not really, and certainly not entirely. The greatest predictor of physician satisfaction is our decision to make it so. To be driven by values, purpose, and making a difference in the patients we treat. It is exhilarating to be a hero, over and over again all day long. To heal, to touch, to care, to make others better…who in the world has the opportunity to do that 25 times a day? Medicine is far from perfect, but life is far too short to spend precious time dismantling and complaining about one of the greatest professions known by anyone. The greatest thing that medicine has to offer is simply there for the taking, requiring only that we slow down enough to find it again, or maybe even to see it for the first time. There is no doubt; we can receive the amazing gift of a brilliant career with the simple offering of our commitment to others.

If you have taken the time to read this book, I know you feel the same way.

A Case Study

THE SHARP HEALTHCARE JOURNEY TO EXCELLENCE

In 2000, Sharp HealthCare, led by CEO Michael Murphy, was considered the health care leader of San Diego. We were a large, successful integrated health care delivery system made up of seven hospitals and three affiliated outpatient medical groups, with over 14,000 employees and 2,600 affiliated physicians. In an effort to assess the state of operations and service within the organization, over 100 focus groups were organized involving patients, staff, and physicians to answer this question: *How are we doing?* How are we doing as an employer for our staff? How are we doing as a place to practice medicine? How are we doing as a place to receive care? The results were very surprising and disturbing to the leadership of a very successful and prideful organization. Despite our "success," the staff, patients, and physicians said we were "fine," "nothing special," and had little exceptional to report. Being "acceptable" was not the ambition of Sharp HealthCare.

Status quo was not okay. Sharp HealthCare was committed to earning the long-standing loyalty of patients, staff, and physicians. Mike Murphy and his leadership team were committed to act decisively on the newfound data. A cross-country search was undertaken to find the most qualified experts to help us change the direction, service, operations, and culture of Sharp HealthCare.

After extensive research and due diligence, an agreement was reached with Studer Group, founded by Quint Studer. Studer Group had developed a "road map" to service and operational excellence designed to deliver results. It had validated its organizational transformation process with breathtaking results with some of the best hospitals in the country.

In early 2001, our efforts were launched. Our commitment to be the best was titled the "Sharp Experience," based on the book by B. Joseph Pine II, *The Experience Economy*. The premise of *The Experience Economy* is that today's marketplace and customer decision making are no longer driven by service alone. "Good service" can be found in nearly every industry. Service had become a commodity, and it was no longer sufficient to drive customer loyalty. It is now the customer "experience" that keeps people coming back. Starbucks is a coffee experience created by the smells, the service, the facility, the colors, the tables, the cups, and the trademark Starbucks logo. The exact same coffee, served at a different place, just wouldn't be the same. Starbucks has taken the ultimate commodity, the coffee bean, and created an empire driven by creating the customer experience.

The Sharp Experience was founded on creating a health care experience for patients. An experience based upon delivering expert medical care in an environment built upon and committed to doing what's best for the patient. An experience built on kindness and compassion as our organizational identity. An experience dedicated to providing the best and getting the most from our health care workforce. An experience based on respect, trust, and collaboration that would earn lifelong loyalty from our patients. The Sharp Experience was a grass-roots commitment to be the best: the best place to work, the best place to practice medicine, and the best place to receive care.

The Sharp Experience began with the development of leadership training with the creation of the Leadership Development Institute. There was a cultivation of a reward and recognition environment for staff throughout the hospitals and clinics. We engaged measurement of patient satisfaction utilizing the Press Ganey survey tool. The fundamentals of service were trained and implemented on every level. Leaders became accountable for unit performance. Supervisors rounded on staff to capture and recognize the great things that were happening every day, rounded to assure the frontline had the tools and equipment they needed to do their jobs, and rounded to assure our must-have behaviors were happening at the patient interface.

The hospital system had success. Patient satisfaction rose from the 17th percentile nationwide to above the 70th percentile. Employee satisfaction improved and nurse turnover reduced to approximately 10 percent, nearly half the state average. Physician satisfaction in our main Sharp Metropolitan Campus climbed to the 95th percentile as measured by Press Ganey, and we were voted the "Best Place to Work" in San Diego by the *San Diego Business Journal* for two consecutive years. Additionally, Sharp was recognized as the number one integrated health care delivery system in the state of California, while enjoying the most successful financial performance in our 50-year history. A new main hospital construction is now underway, and significant investments have been made in state of the art treatment technologies to sustain our marketplace leadership position. The commitment to excellence is working and the road map we have engaged has been validated by undeniable measures.

For the first 18 months following the launch of the Sharp Experience, the medical group administration worked very hard to train leaders, round for outcomes, and implement service standards that resulted in moderate organizational improvement. To this point, physicians were not engaged and did not participate in this administrative effort. Despite these good faith systemic efforts within the medical group, results were slower to materialize compared to our hospital counterparts.

The intrinsic problem of engaging in broad organizational medical group change without direct and timely partnership with physicians was becoming apparent. Our staff, who works all day, every day with our physicians, began to wonder why physicians, the clinical leaders, were not yet visible participants in the Sharp Experience. Our employee satisfaction surveys returned with a priority index reflecting that the most important and most troubling issue for our staff was physicians not engaging in behavior consistent with service excellence. The sustainability of behavioral training and cultural change was becoming compromised since our staff did not believe physicians were modeling the behaviors for which they were accountable. Our staff would rise only as high as our physicians.

Our physician board of directors for the medical group made the decision that the time had come to bring the Sharp Experience to the physicians. In November of 2002, I received a call from my medical director, Donald Balfour, MD, who asked that I be pulled from a patient room to receive his message personally. He then asked me if I was sitting down. He had my attention. "How would you like to be the physician Fire Starter for the Sharp Experience?" he asked. I had no idea what a physician Fire Starter was, so I asked Dr. Balfour, "What's a physician Fire Starter and what would I be doing?" He paused, "We want you to bring the Sharp Experience to the physicians." I was honored to be asked, but terrified of the assignment. First, I knew next to nothing about what the Sharp Experience really was, and second, how in the world would I begin to engage a group of 300 physicians, spread out over 12 clinics and 40 miles, in a commitment to changing how we deliver health care?

I accepted the position of physician Fire Starter, knowing almost nothing about how I would begin to drive and change physician behavior, but knowing in my heart and mind that engaging and leading physicians was going to be fundamental to the success of the Sharp Experience and the success of the organization.

First, I had to equip myself to lead this effort. I read every article and book I could get my hands on in regards to patient satisfaction, physician satisfaction, leadership, and what needs to be done to create physician behavioral change. I attended conferences, including "Taking You and Your Organization to the Next Level" by Quint Studer, and a number of physician leadership training institutes to better learn the predictors of organizational and physician performance.

Next, I met with our physician board of directors to create a common vision of the critical physician role to improve health care guided by the principles of the Sharp Experience. Leadership support from our physician board was crucial to my ability to have credibility and influence with our medical group physicians.

Initially, we launched our physician engagement by conducting a two-hour training program for physicians titled, "The Physicians' Role in the Sharp Experience." We provided prescriptive guidance in terms of how physicians treat patients, staff, and colleagues in a performance-driven organization, committed to exceptional care. We made the case for service excellence as a foundational effort to the success of our group. We created the "burning platform" for why this must be done by sharing our comparative data profiling where we stood compared to our peer medical groups.

As we began to move forward, it became apparent that a number of our physicians were struggling as we began to profile patient satisfaction as a priority physician performance indicator. We implemented physician coaching where individual physicians were contacted and coached one-on-one, providing simple tools based upon the patient satisfaction data and patterns of patient responses in the Press Ganey survey.

We developed an electronic e-mail training process called "Acts of Excellence" sent to all physicians every several months to remind physicians of the prescriptive tactics and behaviors that make a difference for patients.

We implemented the physician code, which is a board-approved outline for how physicians within our organization treat staff, patients, and colleagues. It is now a part of the physician employment handbook and is used for physicians' orientation for new members to our group. We made behavioral expectations clear as physicians joined our organization.

We developed and implemented physician behavioral standards (the "physician pledge"), signed by our physicians and all new hires to continue to align physicians' behavior to organizational objectives. If we wanted to sustain our reputation of excellence in the community, it was important that all physicians engage behavioral competencies as an expectation.

We realized that training helped physicians provide better care and service to patients, but we also realized that it was something that had to be continual and often. Physician training modules were conducted by site over lunch hours, reviewing tactics to improve organizational performance and patient satisfaction through physician behaviors.

Patient satisfaction data was provided to physicians on a quarterly basis through our "physician performance dashboard," a simple, one-page electronic summary of patient satisfaction and national percentile rank for each of the questions patients are asked about care physicians provide. We found the profiling of the data brought about a receptiveness to change and specificity to what physicians needed to do differently.

As we disseminated comparative patient satisfaction data to physicians, we found several vocal physicians in protest of the tool, the sample sizes, and the fact that their patients were richer, poorer, younger, older, and sicker than anyone else's. We listened to these physicians and modified our approach based on their input. We created a standard for a minimum annual number of surveys that would represent a significant sample with predictive value. We began to use specialty-specific comparative data that preempted the apples to oranges argument brought forth by specialty physicians. We brought Press Ganey experts on site to speak with our physician leadership so that we could understand the science behind the measurement. In the end, the minority physician protests created minimal pause for our efforts and we didn't flinch or lose momentum when vocal protests arose.

We gave physicians further guidance and training by providing each of our physicians a "Physician Guide to Service Excellence." The guide was a 30-page, evidence-based manual of behaviors and tactics that improve performance for every element of the patient encounter.

Our physician leadership increased the amount of income at risk for patient satisfaction, beginning to align income with physicians' performance.

We recognized physicians, holding a physician awards dinner, inviting our 20 highest performing physicians to a dinner whose sole purpose was to thank them for the extraordinary work they do for our medical group. We developed a physician pillar award system, where several physicians, nominated by their peers, were recognized for going "above and beyond." Their stories were told at physician staff meetings where they received a round of applause as well as a check for $1,000. Our medical director now dedicates a portion of all of our physician staff meetings to recognizing and thanking physicians in our group who have done something exceptional for the medical group.

Through our journey, we have become a better medical group. Our quality indicators rank us in the top 1 percent in the state of California. Our physician satisfaction has climbed for four consecutive years. We are more financially successful as a medical group than we ever have been. Over 15 percent of our physicians are above the 95th percentile for patient satisfaction. We have implemented advanced patient access throughout our primary care departments, and we have implemented an electronic health record across all regions.

More importantly, physicians are becoming engaged in the prospect of clinical and practice success through providing exceptional care and service to patients. We showed them the vision, provided the tools and training, measured their progress, coached those who struggled, created standards of conduct, and recognized physicians for their efforts. We continue on our mission to become the best, and the road has been cleared through the support, leadership, and engagement of physicians.

BIBLIOGRAPHY

1. Morrow RW, Gooding AD, Clark C. 1995. "Improving Physicians' Preventive Health Care Behavior through Peer Review and Financial Incentives." *Journal of Family Medicine* 4(2): 165-1699.
2. Tufano J, Conrad DA, Sales A, Maynard C, Noren J, Kezirian E, Schellhase KG. 2001. "Effects of Compensation Method on Physician Behavior." *The American Journal of Managed Care* 7(4): 363-373.
3. Tufano J, Conrad DA, Sales A, Maynard C, Noren J, Kezirian E, Schellhase KG. 2001. "Effects of Compensation Method on Physician Behavior." *The American Journal of Managed Care* 7(4): 363-373.
4. Gesensway, Deborah. "Groups Revising Physician Pay to Survive Managed Care." *American College of Physicians Observer*, December 1996.
5. Deutschman, Alan. "Change or Die." *Fast Company*, May 2005, http://www.fastcompany.com/magazine/94/open_change-or-die.html.
6. Donabedian A. 1998. "The Quality of Care. How Can It Be Assessed?" *The Journal of American Medical Association* 260: 1743-1748.
7. Guldvog B. 1999. "Can Patient Satisfaction Improve Health among Patients with Angina Pectoris?" *International Journal for Quality in Health Care* 11: 233-240.

8. Marquis MS, Davies AR, Ware J.E. 1983. "Patient Satisfaction and Change in Medical Care Provider." *The Journal of Medical Care* 21: 821-829.

9. Tandberg, LR, 1984. "Drugs as a Reason for Nursing Home Admissions." *American Health Care Association Journal*, 10: 20.

10. N, Fanale JE, Kronholm P, April 1990. "The Role of Medication Noncompliance and Adverse Drug Rections in Hospitalizations of the Elderly." *Archives of Internal Medicine* 150(4): 841-845.

11. Merck Manual of Diagnosis and Therapy, Section 22. Clinical Pharmacology. Chapter 301. Factors Affecting Drug Response.

12. Merck Manual of Diagnosis and Therapy, Section 19. Pediatrics. Chapter 258. Drug Treatment in Newborns, Infants, and Children.

13. *The Third Report of the Expert Panel on Detection, Evaluation, and Treatment of High Blood Cholesterol in Adults (Adult Treatment Panel III, or ATP III)* (2002) 106: 3359-3366.

14. Murphy J, Coster G. 1997. "Issues in Patient Compliance." *Drugs* 54(6): 797-800.

15. Rhodes KV, Vieth T, He T, et al. 2004. "Resuscitating the Physician-Patient Relationship: Emergency Department Communication in an Academic Medical Center." *Annals of Emergency Medicine* 44: 262-267.

16. Cropley, Carrie. 2003. "The Effect of Health Care Provider Persuasive Strategies on Patient Compliance and Satisfaction." *American Journal of Health Studies.*

17. Heisler M, Bouknight RR, Hayward RA, Smith DM, Kerr EA. 2002. "The Relative Importance of Physician Communication, Participatory Decision Making, and Patient Understanding in Diabetes Self-Management." *Journal of General Internal Medicine* 17: 243-252.

18. Misselbrook D. 1998. "Managing the Change from Compliance to Concordance." *Prescriber* 9(8): 23, 26, 28, 33.

19. SPSS White Paper, 1996. Using Satisfaction Surveys to Achieve a Competitive Advantage.
20. American Hospital Association Reality Check II. 1998, AHA.
21. "Reducing Malpractice Risk through More Effective Communication." *The American Journal of Managed* Care (1997) 3(4): 649-653.
22. "The Doctor-Patient Relationship and Malpractice: Lessons from Plaintiff Depositions." *Internal Medicine* (1994) 154:1365-1370.
23. Stelfox, Ghandi, Orav, Gustafson. 2005. "The Relation of Patient Satisfaction with Complaints against Physicians and Malpractice Lawsuits." *The American Journal of Managed Care* 10: 1126-1133.
24. Bovberg, Petronis. 1994. "The Relationship Between Physicians' Malpractice Claims History and Later Claims: Does the Past Predict the Future?" *Journal of American Medical Association* 272: 1421.
25. Hickson G, Federspiel C, Pichert J, et al. 2002. "Patient Complaints and Malpractice Risk." *Journal of American Medical Association*: 2951-2957.
26. Hickson, Clayton, Entman, Miller, Githens, Whennen-Golstein, Sloan. 1994. "Obstetricians' Prior Malpractice Experience and Patients Satisfaction with Care." *Journal of American Medical Association* 272(20): 1583-1597.
27. Levinson, Roter, Mullooly, Dull, Frankel. 1997. "Physician-Patient Communication. The Relationship with Claims among Primary Care Physicians and Surgeons." *Journal of American Medical Association* 277(7): 553-559.
28. Roter, Hall, Kern, et al. 1995. "Improving Physicians' Interviewing Skills and Reducing Patients Emotional Distress." *Internal Medicine* 155: 1877-1884.
29. *American College of Surgeons (ACS) Surgery: Principles and Practice* (Online). 2002.
30. "Disruptive Behavior and Clinical Outcomes: Perceptions of Nurses and physicians." *The American Journal of Nursing* (2005) 105(1): 54-64, 64-65.

31. Bertakis KD, Roter D, Putnam SM. 1991. "The Relationship of Physician Medical Interview Style to Patient Satisfaction." *The Journal of Family Practice* 32: 175-181.

32. Larsen KM, Smith CK. 1981. "Assessment of Nonverbal Communication in the Patient-Physician Interview." *The Journal of Family Practice* 12: 481-488.

33. Davis MS. 1968. "Variations in Patients Compliance with Doctors Advice: An Empirical Analysis of Patterns of Communication." *The American Journal of Public Health and the Nation's Health* 58: 274-288.

34. Marvel MK, Epstein RM, Flowers K, Beckman HB. 1999. "Soliciting the Patient Agenda: Have We Improved?" *Journal of American Medical Association* 281: 283-287.

35. Harrigan J, Rosenthal R. 1983. "Physicians Head and Body Positions as Determinants of Perceived Rapport." *The Journal of Applied Social Psychology* 13: 496-509.

36. Wasserman RC, Inui TS, Barriatua RD, Carter WB, Lippincott P. 1984. "Pediatric Clinicians Support for Parents Makes a Difference: An Outcome-based Analysis of Clinician-Parent Interaction." *Pediatrics* 74: 1047-1053.

37. "The Effects of Physician Empathy on Patient Satisfaction and Compliance." *Evaluation & the Health Professions* (2004) 27(3): 237-251.

38. Mazzuca SA, Weinberger M, Kurpius DJ, Froehle TC, Heister M. 1983. "Clinician Communication Associated with Diabetic Patients Comprehension of their Therapeutic Regimen." *Diabetes Care* 6:347-350.

39. Robbins JA, Bertakis KD, Helms LJ, Azari R, Callahan EJ, Creten DA. 1993. "The Influence of Physician Practice Behaviors on Patient Satisfaction." *Journal of Family Medicine* 25.

40. Keers, JC, Groen H. Sluiter WH, Bouma J, Links TP. June 2005. "Cost and benefits of a multidisciplinary intensive diabetes education programme." *Journal of Evaluation in Clinical Practice* 11(3): 293-303.

41. Comstock LM, Hooper EM, Goodwin JM, Goodwin JS. 1982. "Physician Behaviors that Correlate with Patient Satisfaction" *Journal of Medical Education* 57: 105-112.
42. Stewart JE, Martin JL. Summer 1979. "Correlates of patients' perceived and real knowledge of prescription directions." *Contemporary Pharmacy Practice* 2(3): 144-8.
43. Centre for Reviews and Dissemination. 2002. Information –only Patient Education Programs for Adults with Asthma. Cochrane Database of Systematic Reviews.
44. Greenfield, Kaplan, Ware et al. 1988. "Patients Participation in Medical Care." *Journal of General Internal Medicine* 3: 448-457.
45. Heisler, Bouknight, Hayward, Smith, Kerr. "The Relative Importance of Physician Communication, Participatory Decision Making and Patient Understanding in Diabetes Self-care." *Journal of General Internal Medicine* 17(4): 243-252.
46. Braddock, Edwards, Hasenberg, Laidley. 1999. "Informed Decision Making in the Outpatient Practice: Time to Get Back to Basics." *Journal of the American Medical Association* 282(24): 2313-2320.
47. Alexy. 1985. "Goal Setting and Health Risk Reduction." *Nursing Research* 34 (5): 283-288.
48. "How Satisfied Are Physicians and Patients When Medical Groups Control Access to Care?" Grant Result, Utilization Management Effects on Physician/Patient Satisfaction, June 1996.
49. Hickson GB, Federspiel CF, Pichert JW, Miller CS, Gauld-Jaeger J. 2002. "Malpractice Risk and Patient Complaints." *Journal of the American Medical Association* 287(22): 2951-2957.
50. Stoller, Gary. 2005. Companies give front-line employees more power. *USA Today*, 26 March.
51. The American Medical Association (AMA) Policy: H-140.913. Disruptive Physician.

52. Buchbinder SB, Wilson M, Melick CF, Powe NR. 2001. "Primary Care Physician Job Satisfaction and Turnover." *The American Journal of Managed Care* 7(7): 701-713.

53. Williams ES, Konrad TR, Linzer M, McMurray J, Pathman DE, Gerrity M, Schwartz MD, Scheckler WE, Douglas J. 2002. "Physician, Practice, and Patient Characteristics Related to Primary Care Physician Physical and Mental Health: Results from the Physician Worklife Study." *Health Services Research* 37(1): 121-143.

54. "Happiness and Humour. A Medical Perspective." *Australian Family Physician* (2001) 30(1): 17-19.

CHAPTER TWO

HEALTHCARE FLYWHEEL

Throughout my travels, I have found that most health care organizations are good. In fact, about 85 percent of patients in the average hospital rank care as good or very good (or say they are satisfied or very satisfied with their care). However, sometimes that is exactly the problem. Feeling "good enough" is often the biggest barrier for an organization in moving to the next level. There may be no sense of urgency.

The challenge, then, is how to move from good to great (and great to greater) so we can sustain the gains and take our success to another level. Sometimes when I ask hospital CEOs how their RN turnover is, they'll say, "Not bad. We're within the state average." I think that in health care, at times, we work at the middle. But we can't afford to do that. We must aim to be the very best.

Since the inception of Studer Group, we've been fortunate to help guide this journey at some of the very finest organizations in the world. They are truly leaders in their field. Yet, they want to get even better. Increasingly, I notice that it is most often the leaders at great organizations who are most committed to further improvement.

Those who succeed do so because their commitment flows from the right reasons: They want to provide better care for patients, a better workplace for employees, and a better place to practice medicine for physicians.

It all starts with a commitment to **Purpose, Worthwhile Work and Making a Difference.** These are the values that rest at the core of the journey and at the hub of the Healthcare Flywheel[SM]. I've met many, many health care professionals, and nearly all of them say they are driven by these core values. This is why most of us went to work in health care in the first place—and likely the reason why you are reading this book. (See? The good always want to get better.)

HEALTHCARE FLYWHEEL[SM]

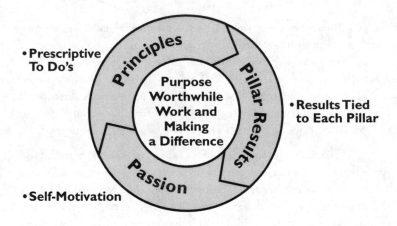

The Healthcare Flywheel shows how organizations can create momentum for change by engaging the passion of their employees to apply prescriptive actions guided by Nine Principles[SM] of service and operational excellence to achieve bottom-line results. By continually reinforcing how daily choices and actions connect back to these core values at the hub of the Flywheel (purpose, worthwhile work, and making a

26

difference), leaders will reinforce these behaviors and effect change more quickly.

SELF-MOTIVATION

The Flywheel is initially turned by passion. Fortunately, people in health care are passionate and self-motivated. Who but a self-motivated person could hold a dying infant in her arms or witness the death of a patient he has come to care about and still come to work every day for more of the same? Of course, the job description also requires many to work with complex reimbursement, keep current on an ever-expanding array of medications and changing procedures in a 365 day-24/7 work environment. The problem is not motivation. It is the ways in which we unintentionally de-motivate employees.

Imagine, for example, that your boss called you into his or her office. Would your first thought be *Here comes more reward and recognition?*

Let's say you work in facility engineering and the telephone rings. You answer, "Facility engineering. This is Debra. How can I help you?"

And someone says, "Yes, this is the staff in the OR. We were just talking today and wanted to call and let you know the temperature is good. It's very comfortable. Thank you."

Does this happen often in your department?

See . . . in health care we are trained to notice the problem, hone in on the negative variance, react to failing systems, disease, and illness. We are professionally trained to be problem-spotters. To a point, this is a good way to avoid mechanical failures, improve financial operations, and ensure quality clinical care. Unfortunately, noticing the negative does not provide the foundation for a positive work culture. I learned that to create a positive relationship, it takes three positive comments to balance every negative one. I am not suggesting that we stop noticing what's wrong; the goal is to

27

substantially increase our awareness and celebration of all that is right. Indeed, there is much to celebrate in health care today. In chapter 5, I will share prescriptive tools you can use to shift your focus organizationwide to what's working well. This is a critical step in creating the kind of organizational culture that turns the flywheel. Without it, there will be little movement and it will not be possible to sustain the gains that are made.

So in summary, we are fortunate to work with so many who have passion for what they do. But it's important that we don't unwittingly sap this innate self-motivation. Once we successfully engage employees on our quest for excellence, the Flywheel begins to spin.

PRESCRIPTIVE TO DO'S

These are the techniques, tools, and behaviors that will achieve results under goals that organizations set under Five Pillars of Excellence: People, Service, Quality, Finance, and Growth (see chapter 3). The prescriptive To Do's will be described throughout the following chapters on the Nine Principles of service and operational excellence. I developed these guiding principles to help leaders focus on how to implement actions that will have the greatest impact. They provide a step-by-step road map to getting and sustaining results.

For example, if a leader is discouraged because of high employee turnover, high nursing agency costs, or scheduling challenges, a motivational talk will only serve as a band-aid for the real problem. Instead, I recommend training a leader how to reduce turnover. This will improve morale and get results as described below.

WHAT ARE RESULTS?

When the prescriptive To Do's are implemented, leaders:

- lower staff turnover;

28

166

- raise employee, physician, and patient satisfaction;

- improve service and quality;

- create greater capacity to serve more patients; and

- ensure a healthier bottom line for their organizations.

As employees see the results of their initial efforts, the Flywheel turns faster and momentum builds. This passion fuels more results in a success spiral. Progress toward goals is measured under metrics established under the Five Pillars previously mentioned (People, Service, Quality, Finance, and Growth).

Many leaders ask me, "How can I keep my staff motivated?" I urge them to focus on two things: (1) drive the prescriptive To Do's that are included throughout this book because they bring results, and (2) always connect results back to purpose, worthwhile work, and making a difference. That feeds and strengthens self-motivation.

I find that the most successful leaders understand and organize around Passion, Prescription, and Results because this combination leads all individuals back to the hub of our deep and universal yearning to have purpose, do worthwhile work, and make a difference. In fact, I urge leaders to always connect the actions they ask of their employees back to how they make a difference and serve an important purpose. They need to hear this.

WHAT HAPPENED TO OUR PRIORITIES IN HEALTH CARE?

In 1998, the American Hospital Administration (AHA) asked hospital CEOs what was on their "To Do" list to move their organizations forward. They received 3,700 responses from leaders who ranked their priorities:

1: Upgrading Technology/Information Systems

2: Integrating Delivery System/Forming a Provider Network

3: Developing New Services/Diversifying into Different Business Lines

4: Re-engineering Business Processes

5: Recruiting Physicians

6: Re-engineering Clinical Services

7: Forming a Physician Hospital Organization

8: Controlling Costs

9: Developing a Medical Services Organization

10: Merging/Consolidating

11: Building/Expanding/Renovating

Source: *AHA News*, March 9, 1998. American Hospital Association Leadership Monitor Survey by the HSM Group.

Employees, patients, and physicians never made the CEOs' top ten list.

In fact, when *Modern Health Care Magazine* reported on the study in a May 11, 1998 article, it said that the study found that executives were not walking the talk: "The report concluded that while health care executives say *customer satisfaction* and *employee retention* are the most important aspects of their business, they fail to invest adequately in either."

I believe these leaders have strong core values and are committed to long-term success. It's just so easy to lose focus when we are putting out fires at every turn. I was certainly guilty of that for many years. For instance, training budgets were hard to come by in those days (and still are today). But consistent, quality training and preceptorship are not disposable budget items. As we face historic workforce shortages and so many other obstacles, I believe that well-trained staff and skilled leadership are non-negotiable.

30

I think that the results of AHA's survey were predictive of the challenges we face today. Fast forward to the American College of Healthcare Executives' October 2003 survey, where 58 percent of responding CEOs said personnel shortages were one of their top three concerns. Workforce shortages have required employees and physicians to become a priority for now. But it can't be another quick fix. Employees, physicians, and patients must always be at the top of the organization's To Do list because they drive everything else. That's how we hardwire excellence for the long term.

I know that all leaders want to create the right environment for patients, staff, and physicians. It's just that we get distracted and lost as we are bombarded by new crises. But when we get uncomfortable, our values call us back home. Today, many leaders are being called back home. If you are reading this book, welcome home. If the leaders of your organization purchased this book for you, then you are indeed fortunate to work for an organization committed to purpose, worthwhile work, and making a difference.

It's Still About the Patient

Note from a Nurse Who Attended "Taking You and Your Organization to the Next Level"

> Attending mandatory conferences ranks high on my list of Least Favorite Things to Do. How can "they" ask me to do any more than I already do? I asked myself. There's no time in my schedule. I can think of a million other excuses, but I don't have the time for that either!
>
> So I attended out of obedience, but with a reluctant heart and closed mind. I'm an old nurse. (I could say I am "seasoned" or "experienced," but I just feel old.) I was quite sure I would not learn anything new about how to care for my patients. The thing about us "old" nurses,

though, is that as we age, we forget things. But can we forget the basic and fundamental things? I had.

For me, this Institute was like a stick of dynamite. It blew a hole in the concrete wall of resistance that I had so carefully constructed between change and me. What took years to build was blown apart in minutes. What I thought was a masterpiece was now rubble. Then, there beneath the rubble, I got a glimpse of myself 30 years ago as a wide-eyed new graduate ready to take on the world with my whole career ahead of me.

It was painful to realize how I had forgotten the vows I made as a nurse. When had my heart grown cold and hard? That dynamite explosion could have been fatal. But I didn't die. Instead it felt more like having surgery. My closed mind was opened! My heart of stone was replaced with a heart of flesh! My failing vision is now clearer than it's been in years! And you know what? It's not about me! It has always been and is still about the patient!

Thank you for rekindling the fire of passion and compassion within the heart of this nurse!

Most sincerely,

Susan, RN

FLYWHEEL MOVING BACKWARDS

When I was hired at Baptist Hospital, Inc. in Pensacola, Florida, the flywheel wasn't moving the way people wanted it to. In February 1996, an employee attitude survey had showed that they were deeply unhappy. In fact, the measurement company said they were some of the most unhappy employees they had ever tested.

At most organizations, employees tend to be less satisfied with compensation and benefits and more satisfied in categories such as, "I like my work" and "I like my department." But at Baptist, employees rated their satisfaction very low in 15 out of 18 categories measured.

The scariest thing about that survey was the disparity of results between top managers and supervisors. Supervisors were ranked below average. But Administration was even worse.

Supervisors could say, "Whew! We were rated a negative two, but top management got a negative eight. I'm surprised we were even able to get a negative two since we were dragging them around!"

At Studer Group, we find this isn't unusual in employee satisfaction surveys at many health care organizations, but it is dangerous because it creates a barrier to creating a culture of true teamwork. To me, this signifies a critical need to consistently invest in leadership and management training so employees can have faith in and align their behaviors with those who guide their organizations.

It also isn't unusual to hear of low survey response rates to employee satisfaction surveys either. Only 39 percent of employees bothered to complete the survey at Baptist. It's easy to rationalize that we only hear from the complainers—or that the survey was poorly timed because (insert excuse: "there was a merger then," "it was a busy time of year," etc.). Of course this disappointing data caused pain. No leader wants to have a workplace that isn't good. But at times, denial can be so great that rationalization and excuses just kick in. But I believe employees work very hard to ensure their feedback is accurate. By listening, we can learn about opportunities to become better.

While a number of things may have influenced Baptist's February 1996 survey results, they were really a blessing because they provided a sense of urgency and a platform for change. They were the foundation upon which we worked to build a culture of service and operational excellence.

IT DOESN'T HAVE TO BE THIS WAY

One of the biggest challenges I find in health care is the "we/they" attitude between middle management and administration. This attitude is pervasive with respect to talk about satisfaction surveys, budgets, or salaries.

I was a *we/they* leader. I was a department manager, and I learned how to deliver bad news with the best of them.

"Bob," I'd say, "I went to HR about your pay raise, but they said no," or, "I fought for us on the budget. Here's the best I could do."

Who's the bad guy? Not me. It's Administration—top management. I positioned administration negatively for my own comfort. I didn't do it on purpose. I did it because no one trained me *not* to. As one leader said to me recently at the end of my two-day talk, "It was just so natural that I was unconscious I was even doing it."

Now, what are the chances that any leader is going to get everything he requested in the budget? What are the odds that she is going to come back after the meeting and say to staff, "Unbelievable! We didn't ask for enough! Yep, he thinks we're understaffed."

You just don't hear things like that. I have also seen senior leaders make these excuses . . .

"If I could, I would, but the Board is leaning **heavy** on me on this one."

or . . .

"I'm open to it, but Corporate says no."

When we blame others, we take purpose out of the equation for the employee. Employees want to be aligned with leaders. They want to work beside and for leaders with the right

34

172

purpose and intent. When attendees leave Studer Group's two-day Institute, I ask them to list actions they will take as a result of having attended. The number-one behavior they resolve to change is to "stop blaming administration." Creating and sustaining a culture of excellence is all about the willingness to take individual ownership of problems and opportunities.

This holds true for senior leaders as well. At the very best organizations, the leadership team is completely aligned with respect to objectives, work, and evaluation.

THE HEALTHCARE FLYWHEEL REQUIRES CHANGE

Change, especially in health care, is never easy. What we're talking about involves making adjustments. While changing clinical procedures is easy and familiar, changing leadership techniques is often more difficult and not within our comfort zones. There are many barriers to change, including:

Denial. I was willing to look at labor, Medicare, or Medicaid, but I wasn't willing to look at me.

Rationalization. It's easy to come up with excuses. Pointing to staffing challenges is a favorite.

At Baptist Hospital, Inc. in Pensacola, I was told our high employee turnover was due to the fact that we were a military town. Two years later, when turnover was down substantially, I noticed that we were still a military town. As long as we could blame the military, we didn't try to fix it. Because it wasn't our fault. What could we do? Once we agreed to do away with the rationalization, we were able to look at specific ways to improve employee selection, orientation, and training to ensure the individuals we hired would be successful. We focused on improving employee satisfaction to increase retention. Rationalization is a barrier to solutions.

Blame. At Holy Cross Hospital in Chicago, we blamed the homeless. They'd sit in our ER. And once they were treated, we discharged them back into the cold. Therefore, we explained, they were giving us a low score on patient satisfaction because they probably weren't happy about that.

Then one day, somebody asked, "We send the survey to people's homes, right?"

"Yep."

"Then, how do the homeless get it?"

It's so easy to assign blame.

Uniqueness. Every health care organization is unique in its obstacles and opportunities. Unfortunately, that makes it easy to discount survey satisfaction scores that compare us to peer organizations or organizations nationwide. "We can't be compared because we're different," we say. I call this tendency to explain away our scores "terminal uniqueness." Organization size and location are two of the most common excuses here.

Unwillingness. When I first arrived at Baptist Hospital, I was walking through an administrative work area one day when I met an employee who treated me terribly. Even the other employees were embarrassed. When I got back to Administration, I said, "I just met the *rudest* woman!"

They said, "Oh, you met Mary."

I asked, "Doesn't her behavior and attitude impact other employees?"

They said, "Oh no. They just ignore her."

The problem is that what gets tolerated gets accepted. Let me explain. In order to move your organization to the next level, not everybody will get to make the trip.

A hospital is not a rehabilitation center for wayward staff. Perhaps you're afraid that if you start firing those people, you'll be understaffed. I want to assure you that this won't be the case.

36

The word gets out in departments where low performers and employees with bad attitudes are held accountable. More people want to work there and those that do have higher morale.

One time a nurse leader came up to me and said, "Quint, I have a real problem. My unit is short-staffed. Nobody wants to work there. The work is tough because it's non-stop and we work like crazy. I can't get people to work on my unit. What should I be doing?"

I told her the first thing she should do is stop telling everyone how bad it was to work in her area. "You and your staff are running all over the hospital saying what a terrible place this is to work," I explained. "What nurse wants to go there? It is a self-fulfilling prophecy!" I suggested this nurse leader sit down with her staff and ask, "What do we need to do so this is a good place to work for all of us?" Then I told her to make sure she did it. Use the concept of the mirror decals I described earlier.

In health care, when one bad thing creates another, we call it a death spiral. When you create a great place for staff to work, vacancies will decrease, morale will rise, and the resulting ownership behaviors will translate to better service, quality, financials, and growth. This is a success spiral.

Not Skilled. I believe individuals want to be effective leaders. But they need training. Maybe they don't know how to do it or what to ask for. Maybe they've asked, but have been told no so often that they've stopped asking. Organizations that invest in training live their values by giving employees the skills they need to be successful. In working with hundreds of hospitals, I have found that most organizations don't spend enough time on skill development for leaders. There are no quick fixes. The key is to build the right competencies into each leader so they can be successful. This is a value dividend.

If we allowed an untrained clinician to care for a patient, it would be considered medical malpractice. Since an engaged, aligned workforce is so critical to hardwiring excellence, I believe that not investing in leadership development is the equivalent of organizational malpractice.

In fact, we have found that approximately 65 percent of employees who leave a job do so due to their relationship with their supervisor. We owe it to the patients, families, physicians, and our employees to train leaders. We owe it to the leaders, too.

HI, I WISH I NEVER MET YOU

E-mail sent to Quint Studer after attending Taking You and Your Organization to the Next Level

> Well, I attended your program in June because my patient satisfaction team asked me to attend. I really didn't want to go. I have a fear of flying anyway. Plus, I really don't like customer service training programs.
>
> So I'm sitting in your workshop when I realize that "I'm the man in the mirror." I thought, Wow, let's try it. So I scripted myself, and what do you know? I started having meaningful conversations with staff. I found out what they needed, and got them the tools and equipment to do their jobs. What a difference this is making for me. I have a new-found purpose (and so have the people who work for me).
>
> And yes, I experienced everything you said I would: the push backs, the barriers are all there. I'm dealing with them, but the first one was me. At first I told my Admin team that we should take our time thinking about when and how to implement all this. But now I'm having so much success that I understand the fundamental need to "just do it." Scripting ... hardwiring ... thank you notes ... outcomes orientation. I'm driving everyone crazy. It's really a lot of fun exceeding your patients' expectations. You really connected with me at the CEO level in your talk. Every CEO needs this wake-up call. I finally realized I was not

38

skilled at talking to my employees until I learned from you how to do it.

Thanks,
Paul
Hospital CEO

UNDERSTANDING SOMETIMES FOLLOWS ACTION

In working with many organizations, experience has shown us that one of the most difficult concepts for leaders to accept is that a person might not understand a behavior until *after* they do it. For example, I got a note recently from a nurse leader who said that she'd been rounding for outcomes (a practice we teach) for a while. She characterized the positive results from rounding as "unbelievable." And yet, she said, it was only after she did it, and did it for a while, that she understood. She had to perform the behavior before she could experience the results.

Understanding comes last.

Until a person can see the result from doing a prescribed behavior, it won't make complete sense.

It's all about action. And it must begin with a decision to act.

A man named Ed once asked me, "If there are two frogs on a lily pad and one decides to jump off, how many do you have left?" "One," I answered, anxious to get back to work. But Ed said there were two.

At first, I was concerned about Ed's mathematical abilities, but then he explained. Making a decision and taking action are two separate behaviors. Some people will decide to jump but never do it. Others will act.

For a long time, I was in the former category. I would make decisions and commend myself for making them (like deciding to go on a diet!), but not act. Or not take enough sustained

39

action. I would say that I was going to hold people more accountable, but not actually do it. The following chapters describe recommended actions that have achieved results at hundreds of organizations. I am confident they will work at your organization too. But only if you actually act and continue to act.

YOU CAN ALWAYS GET BETTER

As I've said, it's usually the good who want to get better. When I first met Bill, he was an excellent 30-year CEO at a great Arkansas hospital (now retired). He came with his leadership team to Pensacola, Florida, to learn about our success at Baptist Hospital, Inc.

At the end of the day, I expressed my admiration for his continued commitment to becoming a better leader. In fact, I said, "Bill, you're a much better CEO than me and you've been doing this for over 30 years. What could you take away from a day like this?"

He looked at me and said, *"Spotlight the performers.* I've always had the tendency to shy away from that because I didn't want to hurt anyone's feelings. But when I get back, I'm going to spotlight the performers."

When Bill went back, that's what he did. Since he had one nursing unit that consistently scored high in patient satisfaction, he invited them to a meeting of department managers and directors and explained to all what a great job they had done. He told everyone that when he was out in the community and people told him that their family members had been on that unit, he always felt relaxed because he knew they had received great care.

Within six months, Bill had *all* of his nurse leaders up front at the department head meeting. His action had incentivized every unit to work harder to meet the recognized standard of excellence. I have found that it is important to spotlight the

40

performers, even when it makes others uncomfortable initially. We have to get comfortable with discomfort because we will experience it frequently when we seek to change the status quo. That's why strong leadership requires so much courage.

When that Arkansas hospital's patient satisfaction skyrocketed through the roof, it was my pleasure to travel there and present Bill with one of Studer Group's Fire Starter awards. The room was packed with employees. And Bill, who was a recognized leader in health care with many, many national and state awards to his credit—cried as he accepted that plaque from me. His staff honored him with a standing ovation.

There's something wonderful about doing the right thing for patients and employees. There's also something special about having your employees recognize and appreciate what you've been up to.

You may already work for one of the best organizations in the nation. Or perhaps you are one of the leading professionals in your field. If you are, I suspect you want to get even better. It comes with the territory.

Bill taught me to always be out in the field learning. And to always strive for ways to get better. To look for new tools and techniques to turn the Flywheel faster.

When a hospital creates passion and uses the prescriptive To Do's that are guided by the Nine Principles I will outline, the Flywheel begins to turn with ever-increasing results. As employees increasingly feel a sense of purpose and understand how their behaviors and actions make a difference, anything begins to seem possible. The sky's the limit!

Patients receive better care. Employees take pride in working for such an excellent organization, and they line up to work there. Physicians refer more patients. Revenues increase. Leaders are more equipped to lead. Training is recognized as essential.

And the Flywheel spins.

41

ON THE POWER OF PASSION

Excerpted from March 1999 INC. Magazine *"90-Day Check Up"*
Interview with Quint

Inc.: What sort of rewards and recognition [do you use]?

Quint Studer: Every company has outstanding people. We make heroes of them. One of our nurses, Cyd Cadena, called up a lady who had been hospitalized to see how she was doing at home. She was in a wheelchair, and she was depressed because she didn't have a wheelchair ramp. The family was so busy working on home health care and a whole bunch of other things that they didn't get a chance to put in a ramp. Well, Cyd called our plant-management person, Don Swartz. And guess what Don did? He built a ramp. Don didn't ask, "Can I do it?" I found out about it because the patient called me. Now we tell that story all over the whole organization. What did we tell our people it was OK to do? Break a few rules. Take a few risks. Don is a star. You have to celebrate your legends.

42

RESOURCES

Use these Studer Group Resources to accelerate the momentum of your Healthcare Flywheel℠...

Books

- *Hardwiring Excellence* - Quint Studer helps health care professionals rekindle the flame and offers a road map to creating and sustaining a Culture of Service and Operational Excellence that drives bottom-line results.
- *101 Answers to Questions Leaders Ask* - Quint Studer offers practical, prescriptive solutions to some of the many questions he has received from health care leaders around the country.
- *Practicing Excellence* - Stephen C. Beeson, MD, directly addresses the physician's role in living the principles that lead to organizational excellence.
- *Results That Last* - Quint Studer brings the principles that have transformed many health care organizations to a broader business audience . . . teaching leaders of all stripes to hardwire their companies with the behaviors, tools, and techniques that create a Culture of Excellence. (Coming in 2007)

Videos

- *Hourly Rounding: Improving Nursing and Patient Care Excellence* - The *Hourly Rounding* video/DVD training is an interactive resource to be used with both nursing and ancillary staff and can be used in group training or self-directed learning situations. This tactic improves both patient safety as well as patient satisfaction.

- *HighMiddleLow^SM Performer Conversations* - This video-based coaching product trains leaders to develop a method to re-recruit high performers, continue to develop middle performers, and move low performers "up or out" of the organization.

- *AIDET: Five Fundamentals of Patient Communication* - Acknowledge, Introduce, Duration, Explanation, and Thank You. AIDET is a comprehensive training tool that will enhance communication within your organization. This simple acronym represents how you can gain trust and communicate with people who are nervous, anxious, and feeling vulnerable.

- *Must Haves^SM Video Series* - Implementing the Must Haves will improve bottom-line results, increase volume and decrease length of stay, and improve clinical outcomes, staff retention, and recruitment.
    - *Volume 1: Rounding for Outcomes* - Discover the power of rounding to proactively lead your organization to higher levels of performance.
    - *Volume 2: Employee Thank You Notes* - Gain new insights into the forceful impact a thank you note can make.
    - *Volume 3: Selection and the First 90 Days* - Increase employee retention and ownership by implementing the peer interview process. Includes four video vignettes demonstrating the peer interview process planning

meeting, the interview, the post-meeting, and a 90-day meeting with an employee.

- ○ *Volume 4: Discharge Phone Calls* - Learn how to use discharge phone calls to demonstrate empathy, improve clinical outcomes, learn about the patient's perception of service, and encourage reward and recognition of staff.
- ○ *Volume 5: Key Words at Key Times* - Build positive results by saying and doing things to help patients, families, and visitors better understand what you are doing and why.

Software

- *Discharge Call Manager: Results in Patient Safety and Satisfaction* - Automates the process for making follow-up calls to recently discharged patients.
- *Rounding Manager: Results through Rounding for Outcomes* - Enables health care organizations to capture and monitor operational and performance data in real time.
- *Leader Evaluation Manager: Results through Accountability* - Leaders can enter, access, and share goals and data easily and efficiently. Automates results measurement and drives accountability.
- *Idea Management Software: Results through Innovation* - Easily and quickly accept, track, implement, and reward employee-generated ideas, and tell your staff that you value their opinions and contributions.

Virtual Seminars

- *Engaging Physicians in Your Journey for Service and Operational Excellence Webinar CD* - Quint Studer and Stephen Beeson, MD, share strategies and tools for engaging physicians. This seminar is ideal for all health care leaders, medical executive committees, medical staff leaders, and office leaders.

- *The Baldrige Award: What's in It for Me?* - Paul Grizzell and Debbie Cardello share what it takes to become a Baldrige Award-winning organization. This seminar is ideal for all health care leaders, medical executive committees, medical staff leaders, and office leaders.

- *Tool for Leaders: Rounding Virtual Seminar* - Quint Studer covers issues that leaders often experience when they engage in rounding and discusses tools that can help drive results.

Tool Kits

- *Physician Selection Toolkit* - A clear-cut strategy developed to help you create a reliable, standardized physician selection process that positions your medical group for success.

- *Hospital-Consumer Assessment of Healthcare Providers and Systems (H-CAHPS)* - A toolkit to help hospitals align their actions with the new Hospital-Consumer Assessment of Healthcare Providers and Systems initiative. While many organizations are well prepared, they may benefit from adjustments to specific practices in order to further improve their patients' perception of care.

Institutes

Studer Group Institutes offer a range of learning opportunities for health care organizations beginning their journey to implementing a Culture of Excellence and those looking to create change in a specific area.

- *Taking Your Organization to the Next Level with Quint Studer -* This hands-on session provides the strategies, tactics, and tools necessary to create a cultural transformation within your organization.

- *Nuts and Bolts of Service and Operational Excellence in the Emergency Department* - Built around Studer Group's Nine Principles® and Five Pillars, this session is designed to teach proven processes that align with the goals of your organization to achieve sustainable, measurable results.

- *Excellence in End-of-Life Care* - Learn to apply service, quality, people, financial, and growth prescriptives and specific leadership principles to strategically improve the quality of end-of-life care in your community, adding life to your patients' days when days can no longer be added to life.

- *Rural Partnership Institute* - Addresses the needs and interests of small/rural hospitals and highlights proven best-practices from successful rural hospitals across the country to improve results, increase return on investment, and maximize their human potential.

- *Focusing Nine Principles on Food and Environmental Services* - Focuses on very prescriptive tools and procedures to improve interdepartmental satisfaction with food and environmental services. The session will build on improving quality, employee satisfaction, menu services, and relationships with nurses.

Webinars

Studer Group webinars provide the latest information and tools on topics critical to health care leaders. Each "on demand" hour-long webinar is available during a 90-day period. Go to ***www.studergroup.com*** to see what webinars are currently available.

Speakers

Studer Group Speakers Bureau offers a variety of time-tested presentations by known experts. Each presentation is carefully customized to meet the particular need and interests of your group and is delivered by the expert of your choice.

**Information on all resources is available
at www.studergroup.com.**

ACKNOWLEDGMENTS

Donald Balfour, MD…For his guidance, leadership, and support

Donna Mills…For her persistence and steadfastness to get results

David Spees, MD…For his constant encouragement and honest opinions

Melissa Loughnane…For her incredibly intelligent review of the manuscript

Michael Murphy…For staying the course under all conditions

Phil Yphantides, MD…For his review and input of the first draft

Rick Gessner…For his detailed edits and allowing me to quote him

Sonia Rhodes…For her tireless enthusiasm to drive change

Carole and Bill Beeson…For decades of help and support and an unbiased readthrough

Floyd Loop, MD…For his expert opinion and guidance in the early going

Corey Slavis, MD…For his honest, detailed input and recommendations

Steven Gabbe, MD…For his readership and input

Julie Kennedy, RN…For taking me under her wing

Francesca Funk, LVN…For delivering service excellence to every patient, every time

BG Porter…For his leadership and support to get this done

Bekki Kennedy…For doing everything required to bring this to print

Quint Studer…For his shared, contagious passion to make a difference

About Dr. Beeson

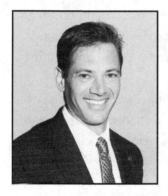

Dr. Stephen Beeson is a nationally recognized presenter who has provided tools and tactics for engaging and training physicians to medical groups and hospitals throughout the country. Dr. Beeson's physician training efforts have focused on providing tactical behaviors to physicians to improve patient care and drive organizational performance through physician engagement, leadership, and excellence by example.

Stephen Beeson is a board certified family medicine physician practicing with Sharp Rees-Stealy Medical Group. In 2002, Dr. Beeson was selected by Sharp HealthCare leadership to serve as the physician Fire Starter for the Sharp Experience, an organizational commitment to service and operational excellence. Dr. Beeson's patient satisfaction ranks him in the 99th percentile nationwide, and he was voted one of San Diego's best physicians by the San Diego County Medical Society in 2005 and 2006. Dr. Beeson was also a recipient of the Center of Recognized Excellence Award for Individual Service Excellence in 2006.

Dr. Beeson graduated *magna cum laude* from the University of California, where he also completed his medical school and residency training.

Dr. Beeson has authored and developed training programs at site, department, and group-wide levels to over 300 physicians. He has developed and implemented the Sharp Rees-Stealy Physician Pledge, the Physician Performance Dashboard for patient satisfaction, the Physician Guide to Service Excellence, developed the Physician Excellence Award Program, new physician orientation and training, individual physician coaching, physician interviewing and selection processes, and the Acts of Excellence electronic physician training program.

Dr. Beeson is passionate about providing exceptional care to patients and works with Studer Group as a medical advisor and speaker to broaden the difference he can make with physicians across the country. Dr. Beeson articulates a strategic and prescriptive road map to medical organization performance through physician training and engagement in *Practicing Excellence: A Physician's Manual to Exceptional Health Care.*

Index

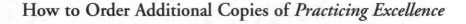

How to Order Additional Copies of *Practicing Excellence*

Orders may be placed:

Online: *www.firestarterpublishing.com* (bulk discounts available)

By phone: 866-354-3473

By mail: Fire Starter Publishing
913 Gulf Breeze Parkway, Suite 6
Gulf Breeze, FL 32561

Practicing Excellence also is available online at *www.amazon.com*.